Words of Praise for *The Right Weigh*

*"It's all here—everything anyone needs
to know and do to lose weight and keep it off
joyfully and healthfully. This book is a treasure!"*

— **Christiane Northrup, M.D.,** the author of *Women's Bodies,
Women's Wisdom* and *The Wisdom of Menopause*

*"America is suffering from an epidemic of obesity,
with no limit in sight.* **The Right Weigh** *offers a way out—
a natural, sane approach that takes into account body, mind,
and spirit. This perspective is vastly needed if we are to
learn how to live in harmony and balance with food."*

— **Larry Dossey, M.D.,** the author of
Reinventing Medicine and *Healing Words*

*"Rena Greenberg hones in on one of the deepest causes
of overweight—our thoughts about it—and helps us to
dismantle those thoughts.* **The Right Weigh** *provides
help that many people have been praying for."*

— **Marianne Williamson,** the author of
The Gift of Change and *A Return to Love*

*"If you do not feel loved, you will find addictive,
self-destructive behaviors to replace the feelings you seek
to experience. Rena Greenberg's guidance can help you to
reparent yourself and nourish the Divine child within you
in ways that will lighten your mind, body, and spirit."*

— **Bernie Siegel, M.D.,** the co-author of *Help Me to Heal*
and the author of *365 Prescriptions for the Soul*

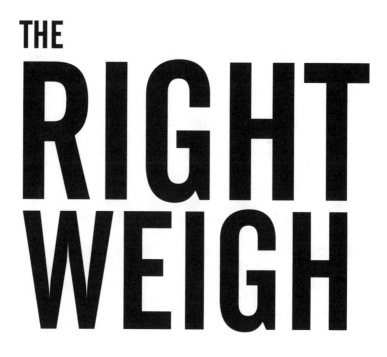

THE
RIGHT
WEIGH

Hay House Titles of Related Interest

Kits by Jorge Cruise

8 Minutes in the Morning®:
A Simple Way to Shed Up to 2 Pounds a Week—GUARANTEED!

8 Minutes in the Morning® to a Flat Belly: *Lose Up to 6 Inches in Less than 4 Weeks—GUARANTEED!*

8 Minutes in the Morning® to Lean Hips and Thin Thighs: *Lose Up to 4 Inches in Less than 4 Weeks—GUARANTEED!*

❖❖❖❖❖❖

All of the above are available at your local bookstore, or may be ordered by visiting:

Hay House USA: **www.hayhouse.com**
Hay House Australia: **www.hayhouse.com.au**
Hay House UK: **www.hayhouse.co.uk**
Hay House South Africa: **orders@psdprom.co.za**

THE
RIGHT
WEIGH

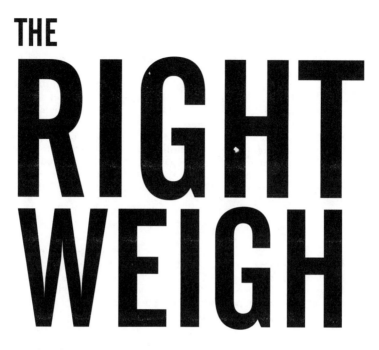

Six Steps to Permanent
Weight Loss Used by More
Than 100,000 People

RENA
GREENBERG

HAY HOUSE, INC.
Carlsbad, California
London • Sydney • Johannesburg
Vancouver • Hong Kong

Published and distributed in the United States by: Hay House, Inc., P.O. Box 5100, Carlsbad, CA 92018-5100 • *Phone:* (760) 431-7695 or (800) 654-5126 • *Fax:* (760) 431-6948 or (800) 650-5115 • www.hayhouse.com • **Published and distributed in Australia by:** Hay House Australia Pty. Ltd., 18/36 Ralph St., Alexandria NSW 2015 • *Phone:* 612-9669-4299 • *Fax:* 612-9669-4144 • www.hayhouse.com.au • **Published and distributed in the United Kingdom by:** Hay House UK, Ltd. • Unit 62, Canalot Studios • 222 Kensal Rd., London W10 5BN • *Phone:* 44-20-8962-1230 • *Fax:* 44-20-8962-1239 • www.hayhouse.co.uk • **Published and distributed in the Republic of South Africa by:** Hay House SA (Pty), Ltd., P.O. Box 990, Witkoppen 2068 • *Phone/Fax:* 27-11-706-6612 • orders@psdprom.co.za • **Distributed in Canada by:** Raincoast • 9050 Shaughnessy St., Vancouver, B.C. V6P 6E5 • *Phone:* (604) 323-7100 • *Fax:* (604) 323-2600

Editorial supervision: Jill Kramer • *Design:* Tricia Breidenthal

Library of Congress Cataloging-in-Publication Data

Greenberg, Rena.
  The right weigh : six steps to permanent weight loss used by more than 100,000 people / Rena Greenberg.
    p. cm.
  ISBN-13: 978-1-4019-0687-0 (tradepaper)
  ISBN-10: 1-4019-0687-7 (tradepaper)
  1. Weight loss. 2. Nutrition. 3. Health. I. Title.
  RM222.2.G722 2005
  613.7--dc22
                                  2005020456

                ISBN 13: 978-1-4019-0687-0
                ISBN 10: 1-4019-0687-7

                08 07 06 05   4 3 2 1
                1st printing, December 2005

                Printed in the United States of America

*This book is dedicated to my Creator,
with the deepest gratitude for unlimited
love and strength—for showing me the higher
way, and for always being there to gently and
mercifully guide me back onto the straight path.*

CONTENTS

PREFACE ●●●●●

How the Right Weigh Program Came About

My wake-up call came when I was 25 and mysteriously started to feel chronically exhausted. Prior to that, I'd been healthy, energetic, and enjoying my youth fully. However, I didn't have any concept of taking care of myself. I was highly addicted to sugar and caffeine in any form—rich carbohydrates, alcoholic beverages, and an unlimited supply of coffee—although I was only about 15 to 20 pounds overweight because I exercised excessively. I certainly didn't know about listening to my body or eating, resting, exercising, and living in a balanced and moderate way.

I went from one doctor to another in search of an answer to my "condition," and tried to will myself back to health with various diets and exercise routines, to no avail. Finally, after being advised by an acupuncturist and a physical-education teacher that my heart rate was irregular, I walked over to the hospital nearest to my home in Park Slope, Brooklyn, certain that there was nothing physically wrong with me. To my surprise, I was whisked right into the ER and told that my heart rate was 30 beats per minute and the only thing keeping me alive was my age.

I was taken directly to the cardiac-care unit, where the chief cardiologist announced that I had the heart of an 80-year-old. Because it was an emergency situation, he attached a temporary pacemaker to my heart through a large vein that originated in my thigh. But before he left for the weekend, he gave strict orders to the resident doctor and the nurses to leave the device shut off so that he could see what would happen to my natural heart rhythm.

Late the next evening, I started to feel extreme pain in my chest that was radiating down my left arm. The resident doctor (who appeared not to have slept in days) took little notice and gave me a drug that caused my ears to ring but had no effect on the pain. After he left the room, my pain grew stronger. The nurse on duty told me that she couldn't go against the doctor's orders and turn the pacemaker on, even though I was begging her to at that point.

I have no idea how much time elapsed, but I do know that the pain grew stronger and stronger, and I was quite certain that I was having a heart attack. There was a pacemaker on my leg, but I didn't know how to turn it on! My prayer to God came naturally for me at that point, as it probably would for anyone in the same position.

What's interesting, in retrospect, is that I did not pray for myself. What came to me in that moment as I sat clutching my heart with both hands, tears streaming down my face, was the strong image of my mother. She's a German Jew and had lived through the Holocaust. She'd already suffered so much loss in her life, yet I knew that my death was the worst thing that could happen to her. So in that moment as I sat up in bed at New York Methodist Hospital, clutching my chest and wracked with pain, I prayed for her: "Dear God, please let me live for my mother. If I die now, it will kill her. Please give me back my life for her." In that instant, the frightened young nurse burst into my room and turned on the pacemaker against the doctor's orders, and of course my pain subsided.

The next day, the chief of cardiology implanted a permanent pacemaker into my chest, and I was discharged a week later. I know that had it not been for the sudden action of that nurse, who I'm certain was guided by God, I wouldn't be alive today.

Our minds can't understand miracles, but we can certainly be in awe of their occurrence. Following that experience, I committed myself to learning about the power of love. I have no doubt that it was my care for my mother—and God's love for both of us—that kept me alive.

Pain is a strong motivator, and being sick had brought me a lot of it. When I got out of the hospital, I felt dedicated to changing my old, destructive ways. I was determined to find true health of mind, body, heart, and spirit, so I learned about the importance of balance for the physical body—the need for adequate rest and physical activity—as well as how crucial it is to eat a variety of whole, unprocessed foods.

I studied the reality of sugar addiction and how to overcome it once and for all, as well as the immense power of the mind to transform the way we all see ourselves and the way we relate to our environment. But by far my greatest discovery was the Higher Intelligence that resides in our hearts. This ocean of Divine Love, provided by our Creator, can help us evolve beyond our wildest dreams, as long as we're willing to surrender to and open up to this force.

After regaining my health, I went on to study psychology, hypnosis, biofeedback, neuro-linguistic programming, and many other healing modalities. By combining all of these systems, I developed the Right Weigh program, which can help you reach and maintain your ideal weight. I know this method works because I've not only used it to transform my own life, I've also guided more than 100,000 people through it in private sessions and at weight-loss seminars in over 70 hospitals and 100 corporations since 1989.

As I was conducting weight-loss seminars in medical centers throughout Florida, Michigan, and New York, I met many people who'd tried every method possible to lose weight. I heard tragic stories of men and women who'd triumphed and dropped many pounds, only to gain them back shortly thereafter. As I listened to their stories and felt the heartache and desperation that they were experiencing, I realized that there really was no road map out there for people trying to lose weight permanently.

Sure, there are scores of books on diets (and most likely there will continue to be), but if you're picking up *this* volume, I'm willing to bet that the problem isn't that you don't know what a sensible meal plan is. My guess is that you understand that exercise is crucial for permanent weight loss and are aware whether you're using food in an unhealthy way—such as engaging in overeating, bingeing, snacking, or emotional eating. That's why I'm not going to tell you exactly what to eat or how to exercise (although I will give you guidance on creating an eating and exercise plan that works for you). Instead, I'm going to focus on helping you change yourself on the inside so that sticking to your plan isn't an impossible chore, but a simple habit that feels natural to you . . . which I know might sound like an ambitious plan.

You may be wondering what you can do to change your behavior when you've tried so hard to be in control of your life and your eating habits but still haven't been able to lose the weight and keep it off. Where will you find the strength to try again? How can you keep from simply giving up when you feel so weak around food? If only it didn't taste so good—and if only exercise weren't so difficult, tedious, and time-consuming!

Without the proper tools, the task of losing weight can seem insurmountable—especially using the methods you've tried in the past. You know that diets don't work, you realize that they're a psychologically temporary situation, and you've found out how difficult it is to stick with them over the long haul.

Dieting isn't the answer, and neither are expensive fitness centers. It's not that you need more willpower; instead, you need to access your greatest strength and reclaim your life. Once you truly understand how your subconscious works, you can begin to reprogram your own mind so that you'll automatically start behaving in ways that lead to the result you so desire.

The Right Weigh will teach you how to harness the power within your deeper mind, heart, and spirit to help you achieve the health and body that you deserve to have—and stop using food to fill a void.

It's truly a privilege to share with you the knowledge that has had such a profound effect on my life. I started off just interested in getting my health and my body back—wanting to lose weight, feel good, and have energy. My personal journey has led me beyond those early goals to a life of more freedom, fullness, and peace than I could have ever imagined. I want you to know what's possible for you when you commit to living each day inspired by your innate connection to the Divine within you. When you begin to tap in to the greater resources within your very own mind and heart, you can achieve your ideal weight . . . and so much more.

INTRODUCTION

How to Use This Book and Work the Right Weigh Program

This book is divided into two parts. Part I outlines productive eating and lifestyle behaviors that I want you to use throughout your journey, both as you're working the six steps and doing the exercises that are in Part II. This first section teaches you how to finally achieve balance with the foods that you're eating, maintaining health while enjoying your meals to the fullest. You'll also find many ideas for planning ahead, using items that taste good and that are completely satisfying to you.

The changes you'll need to make are simple and easy and can be incorporated into the busiest lifestyle. You'll still be able to enjoy what you eat to the fullest when you select foods that nourish your mind, body, and spirit. Part of being prepared includes incorporating physical activity into your life, stretching your muscles, and working with the stress-reduction methods I'll teach you.

You'll also learn how to handle food addictions, particularly the most common one: sugar. Some of you may not have this problem (or may think that you don't), but I urge you to read this section and consider the possibility that you might have insatiable cravings for certain goodies that are preventing you from losing weight and keeping it off. I'll teach you easy and practical ways to live in the real world, free from the triggers that have kept you stuck in the throes of addiction.

As you read Part II of this book, you'll begin to truly understand why you've had so much difficulty achieving your ideal weight. You'll take a closer look at the conscious and the subconscious mind and the difference between the two. You'll find that in your conscious, rational mind, you're very motivated to live your life at your ideal weight and be healthy and fit. Consciously, you understand that it's possible for you, despite past failures, and you know exactly what you need to do in order to achieve your goal. You recognize that you need to choose smaller portions, eat healthier foods, and increase your activity level.

The success that has eluded you up to this point has nothing to do with a lack of knowledge or not enough motivation or willpower. Rather, it's related to the *subconscious* obstacles that have kept you stuck. These are the voices, images, habits, and beliefs that have you convinced you'll never really change and that you're destined to a life of being overweight and out of control when it comes to eating.

You'll learn about how to get past the challenges of pleasurable associations with the wrong foods and painful impressions about exercise, as well as the unproductive habits of overeating, bingeing, snacking, and emotional eating that you may have developed over time. Using food as a drug to give you energy, sedate you, or fill an inner void has kept you from achieving what you truly want for yourself.

Within Part II, you'll learn about the six steps to permanent weight loss. In Step 1, "Know Your Vision," you'll begin to set a new course for your life—one that's consistent with your deepest heart's desire to be free from food addiction and live your life in greater happiness and harmony with yourself. In Step 2, "Turn to Your Source for Help," I'll help you become consciously aware of the ally you have within yourself: the Divine Love in your very own heart. When you fully connect with this Source of immense love and wisdom, you'll discover for yourself—perhaps for the first time in your life—how alive and creative this energy is. You can then tap in to this immense force of love and creativity to gain control over your life and your eating habits.

Step 3, "Accept Yourself as You Are," is about fully accepting yourself and your life situation as it is in this moment. Yes, you may wish that the circumstances were different, but until you say yes to what *is,* nothing is very likely to change. But once you break the cycle of harsh, negative self-talk, new possibilities that are consistent with what you truly desire will begin to open up for you.

Step 4, "Break Free from Obstacles," will help you look at what's held you back in the past and learn how to overcome these road-blocks on your journey to a healthy, fit body. Step 5, "Reprogram Your Subconscious Mind and Create Your Future," is about using neuro-linguistic programming and self-hypnosis to change your mind and your future to make it consistent with your deepest longing.

Finally, Step 6, "Letting Go of the Past," will give you an opportunity to acknowledge your mistakes, stop beating yourself up for them, and simply move forward. In order to step into a greater future, it's necessary to fully let go of what was and forgive yourself. Step 6 will guide you to release any of the old burdens that you may be carrying (such as guilt or shame for the way you've treated your body), and fully embrace the new life that awaits you.

Please keep in mind, however, that while the inner work of the six steps in Part II is absolutely crucial for losing weight, you also must do the outer work outlined in Part I, consistently behaving in ways that lead to your goals. For instance, if you pray all day long for help in losing weight but never change the way you eat or engage in any physical activity, you clearly won't see much visible progress.

The purpose of your deep, heartfelt prayer is to connect with your greatest Source of guidance, and with practice, you can learn to access your inner wisdom readily. When you're connected in this way, you'll have the motivation to follow through with the actions that are in alignment with your goal. And more than that, you'll also have a deep knowing about what you need to do in order to live at your ideal weight and be healthy in mind, body, and spirit.

Once you receive guidance about your own personal weight-control plan from your deep inner wisdom, you must commit to following the advice that you've been given. This plan is going to be unique to you. As your commitment to yourself and living your life to a fuller potential is strengthened, you'll naturally find yourself making the necessary changes in your behavior. You'll start to actually enjoy and appreciate healthier dishes, and it will become easier to leave food on your plate and listen to the hunger signals from within. Your sensitivity to the effects that the meals you're choosing have on your body will become enhanced, and you'll start naturally gravitating toward healthier choices. You'll start to look forward to the time of day when you *get* to exercise, rather than dreading it. The actions that will lead you to your heartfelt, desired outcome will start to spring forth naturally.

As you go through Part II, it will become evident to you what you need to work on in order to reach your desired weight and live a happier and more peaceful life. Maybe you'll need to eliminate certain foods; eat more slowly; drink more water; appreciate the foods you're consuming; or truly love, honor, and nurture your body. As you work through the exercises—and begin taking action using the information and guidance provided in Part I—you'll be able to let go of your past mistakes and move into a beautiful and satisfying future.

The second section of this book begins with Chapter 4, which will explain how to get the most out of the exercises you'll be doing as part of your plan—and there's no cardio or weight lifting involved! I urge you to read this chapter, take in its ideas, and make a firm commitment to work this program for at least 40 days, or approximately six weeks. You'll also find a layout of what you'll be doing all that time, which I suggest you photocopy and place near your calendar or on your wall, where you can look at it every day. Write down the date of each day of the plan so that you don't get confused. (For instance, if you begin the program on January 1, Day 8 would be January 8.)

Each of the chapters describing the six steps is filled with powerful exercises that will stretch you on the inside, where it really counts. By performing these explorations, you'll become aware of your own obstacles and break any unhealthy patterns that are leading to your overweight condition. You'll also be able to access your subconscious mind and reprogram the way you think about yourself and food. No matter how long you've been holding on to obstacles, you'll be able to change the unproductive programming that isn't serving you.

You'll learn how to reconnect with your own deepest truth so that you can gain control of your life and your eating habits. Using these exercises, you'll get in touch with your higher attributes of strength, patience, and compassion for yourself—and you'll no longer need to eat to fill a void of emptiness. Even though you'll be consuming less, you'll feel satisfied.

This regimen is simple, yet the impact it can have on your life is profound. You have nothing to lose—except the weight that's been bogging you down. So give yourself these weeks to discover the truth about what resources actually do live inside of you that you can draw upon.

You'll work on each of the six steps for approximately a week. It's fine to stay with one longer or to repeat a step if you feel that you need more time. This isn't a race; you're permanently changing the way you relate to yourself and food. If you miss a day for whatever reason, don't worry about it—just get right back to doing the exercises. By the time you're finished, you will have developed a new, positive habit of taking time out for yourself every day to access the bountiful treasure within your deeper mind and heart.

Each step has several exercises for you to do. Please practice each of them at least once, and then repeat the ones that you're most comfortable with—the ones that resonate for you. The more you practice them, the greater the benefit you'll receive, and the easier it will become to incorporate the skills into your life. There are a few that you should do every day, however, and you'll find my overview of those at the end of Chapter 4.

My deepest heart's desire is to take your hand and lead you from where you are to where you want to go. I want you to experience permanent weight loss, as well as a life filled with joy, gratitude, confidence, and deep satisfaction regarding your weight and the control you have over it. If you just read this book from cover to cover, you may find some helpful nuggets. However, to extract the greatest benefit, it's imperative that you actually do the exercises every day. I encourage you to practice them for at least 30 minutes a day for a minimum of 40 days, or approximately six weeks (the program is six weeks because studies show that's about how long it takes to break a habit). Commit yourself to this program because you're worth it! Make it a priority that you refuse to break. Haven't you spent enough of your life in struggle?

As you embark on this journey, know that you already have everything that you need to be successful. You're simply learning how to access and use what you've been given. It's my hope that you'll be inspired to follow through and work the program to create profound change in your life.

Now, before you embark on any journey, it's important to realize that it isn't necessarily going to be a straight path. After all, when an airplane flies from Los Angeles to New York, it's off course much of the time, but the pilot knows the final destination. If he finds himself straying, he's not going to just land in Houston; he's going to get back on track toward New York. You, too, may find yourself veering at times, and that's okay, because you'll know where you're going and can easily refocus.

You have an extremely important vision for yourself: to live your life as a person who's healthy, fit, at your ideal weight, and in control. Without a clear vision of where you're going, you can never get there. So the first thing you need to do is choose *your* most compelling goals.

Continue to follow the Right Weigh program and you'll transform your life completely. One day, you'll look back and realize that you truly are different—but now you simply have to take that first step. Don't be afraid to trade in your life tickets for a destination more pleasing than the one you've been headed toward in the past. Most important, enjoy your journey . . . and the many treasures you'll undoubtedly discover along the way.

A PRACTICAL WEIGHT-LOSS APPROACH

PART I

CHAPTER ONE

The Basic Components of Weight Loss

More Americans are overweight now than ever before. The myriad of diets, weight-loss clinics, and fitness centers that are available seem to be having no effect on this crisis. If you're like many people, you're concerned about your health, ashamed of your appearance, and uncomfortable in your clothes—yet when it comes to reversing this situation, you've been unable to effect any lasting change.

Right now, you're at a very important juncture, so are you going to continue on the path you've been on, going from one diet to the next, failing to lose the weight and keep it off, and feeling completely frustrated and ineffectual? How long can you continue to begin expensive fitness plans, filled with high hopes and expectations, only to be let down by your own inability to maintain the exercise level you felt so committed to only days or weeks before? Can you continue enduring the nagging guilt associated with eating foods that are poisonous to your system—yet feel completely out of control and powerless when it comes to making permanent change?

If you answered yes to any of the above questions, then perhaps you need to switch tactics.

Where Can You Turn for Answers?

If you're like a lot of people, you've been conditioned to look outward for advice on how to solve the dilemma you face regarding your weight. You probably expect the experts to tell you whether you should be eating butter or margarine; if eggs are a healthful source of protein or a magnet for high cholesterol; and whether you should take up jogging or just stroll through the park. The problem is that every time you turn to a different "expert," you'll get different advice because no one approach is going to work for everyone . . . and it can be overwhelming to have so many choices.

How can you avoid becoming completely discouraged by the lack of any clear, concise direction? And where can you turn for help in making the necessary, permanent changes in your diet and lifestyle? It's time you started to look in a new direction. Rather than consulting others, turn to a place within yourself that knows what is and isn't best for *you.*

Your Deepest Longing

What does your heart truly desire? Whatever it is, know that you *can* have whatever you want. If, for instance, your deepest longing is to be happy and healthy, in control of your life and your eating habits, living fit and at your ideal weight, and serving the world in the way you were created to do . . . then know that this is not only possible, it's your destiny. If such a goal feels unattainable to you (or has felt that way up until now), realize that it's because there hasn't been a road map for you to get from where you are to where you want to go.

You're going to journey to a place where you can be at peace with yourself and your weight, enjoy the food that you're given, and naturally choose and desire the types of dishes and the serving sizes that support your health and vitality. You'll be able to focus on what you're here to give in your precious lifetime, rather than criticizing yourself or acting self-destructively. This state of peace and fulfillment exists within your heart: It's your soul's longing to live life fully. By following the six steps of the Right Weigh program, you'll deepen your contact with the wise, loving Source inside you and begin to live your life the way you were meant to.

Although the exercises in Part II focus on making internal changes to truly embrace the life that you wish to create, it's important to realize that you can spend your entire time on Earth in prayer and meditation, but if you don't take action and change your activity level and the way you eat, the numbers on the scale won't budge. The six steps of this program are designed to help you focus all of your energy and life force on achieving the vision you desire for yourself: living healthy, happy, fit, and at your ideal weight. You'll also strengthen your connection to the Source of life, which is always available to help you.

The Equipment You'll Need

Before you begin the Right Weigh 40-day, six-step program, you'll need to gather the following supplies:

— **Food diary:** You can use a small, blank notebook that you'll fill in with the appropriate categories listed on page 32, or you can make copies of that example. Whichever one you choose, it should be small and flexible enough for you to carry around with you wherever you go, such as in your purse or pocket.

— **Index cards:** You'll need a package of 3" x 5" blank white index cards.

— **Tape recorder and blank tapes:** Recording the exercise instructions in Part II and playing them back as you rest in a comfortable position will benefit you much more than simply reading through them. You'll need a tape recorder and about a dozen blank tapes with labels.

— **Permanent-weight-loss journal:** Using a journal is an excellent way to work through the exercises in this book. When you take the time to write things down rather than just think of them, it can make a huge difference. You see, this seemingly simple act of writing things down has an enormous impact on the subconscious part of your mind. By noting the reasons that you're absolutely committed to losing that excess weight once and for all—and keeping it off forever—you're impressing those new, productive thoughts on your deeper mind.

Also, when you use a journal, you'll have a chance to go back and look at what you've written, reviewing your goals. Buying a beautiful book for this task gives you a tactile and visual reminder that you value what you're writing down—that this isn't some annoying chore or homework assignment, but an important record of your self-transformation.

When your conscious and subconscious mind are in harmony with your heart's deepest longing, it becomes much easier to manifest good things in your outer reality.

Let's begin by discovering what actions are essential for you to reverse your condition, achieve your ideal weight, and maintain it for the rest of your life. These beginning chapters will give you a foundation for the transformation you'll experience in the second part of this book.

The Necessary Components of Weight Loss

Why are you overweight? It doesn't matter if you don't think you eat very much or if you walk three times a week: The bottom line is that if you consistently take in more calories than you're burning off, you'll remain overweight, or even gain more.

Everyone overeats at times—but is your behavior a habit or a rare occurrence? If you do overindulge, do you balance that by consuming less for a while or increasing your activity level? Maintaining an ideal weight over time is always achieved through these basic components: the amount of food you eat and your ability to burn those calories. In this chapter, you'll get an overview of the most important things to remember about each of these points.

Are You Eating Too Much?

Many overweight people tell me that they don't eat very much. Often, however, they're doing it unconsciously, as if the calories don't count if they're standing up, on vacation, driving a car, and so on. Being oblivious to hidden sources of calories—such as plopping Bac-Os and high-fat dressing on a salad or eating huge portions just to get your money's worth—doesn't stop them from putting on weight.

I was once listening to a program on weight control, and the speaker said something that shocked me: He said that there were no overweight people in the concentration camps. Then I realized that although it was in poor taste, what he said was true—that is, when you don't eat, you aren't going to gain weight. (One exception to that could be if you're on certain medications that are causing you to gain.)

Have you just given up on changing yourself because of your belief that no matter what you do it won't make a difference . . . because of hormones, medications, or metabolism? Don't worry—this is quite common. I applaud you for picking up this book, which is a way of telling yourself that there are some things that are under your control, and they're what you can focus on. While these problems can certainly be discouraging, I've seen people on thyroid medication and other prescriptions that were slowing down their metabolisms lose weight by using the methods in this book simply because they could still control things to a degree by changing their eating habits and increasing their activity level. If this is your situation, you may not lose as quickly as someone who doesn't have those impediments, but you can still reduce by following this program.

If you start eating smaller portions, then you can continue to eat the foods that you grew up with, appreciate, and enjoy. By taking in less, you'll naturally start reducing. A few ways you might do this include:

- Leaving food on your plate, even if you feel resistance. If you don't want to waste it, wrap it up to eat later when you're actually hungry.

- Beginning to eat half the amount that you normally would. Start with small portions, and don't go back for seconds.

- Establishing the habit of pushing your plate away before you feel full so that you give your brain time to register that your stomach is satiated. Don't overeat! Even the healthiest foods can do damage if consumed in excess.

- Chewing slowly and enjoying each bite. This will help you eat less, stopping you before you've overfilled your stomach. Keep checking with your belly to see if you're full. (Slowing down will also help you notice the textures and tastes of food.)

Counting Calories

If calorie counting works for you, that's fine—get a calorie book and calculate how many you'd have to eat in a day to lose one pound a week, keeping in mind that it takes 3,500 calories to gain or lose a pound. If you're choosing this approach, write down everything you eat in order to keep track of it. If you continually take in fewer calories than you're burning off, you're going to lose weight.

There's nothing intrinsically wrong with this method, particularly if you don't want to restrict the types of foods you eat (which is discussed in Chapter 2). If you believe that you can use a Weight Watchers type of plan and eat a little of everything, including sugary foods, then try it. But if you know yourself and can honestly say that this type of diet has never worked for you, why put yourself through the agony of failure again?

Even if you don't track calories precisely, it *can* be helpful to have an awareness of them so that you can make them count! For example, when you're at a restaurant, you may decide that the day-old bread isn't worth the calories, so you remove it from your sandwich. However, that hot, fresh bagel on Sunday morning might be a wonderful way to use your calories from bread products for the week. This is a more balanced approach than simply eating all bread products at any time you aren't on a diet, and then switching to total restriction and deprivation, even if there's an occasion to really enjoy a moderate treat or you're particularly hungry.

When making your selections, be aware that all calories aren't created equally. Fibrous foods are more filling per unit. For example, 100 calories of raspberries and blueberries is far more satisfying than the same value of fruit juice. The fiber—the skins of fruit or the husks of whole grain—will fill you up.

Enjoy Physical Exercise

Besides cutting back on your portions and choosing healthier foods, increasing your activity level is the best thing you can do for yourself when it comes to taking off and keeping off weight. Not only does it burn calories, but a regular schedule of physical activity will increase your resting metabolism, even when you're sleeping—what a great payoff! On top of that, you'll feel better, have more energy, and reduce your stress level naturally.

Is *exercise* a negative word for you? Does it bring up pictures of aching muscles, tedious workouts, and exhaustion? If so, you'll need to reframe these unproductive associations by starting to think in terms of increasing your activity, and it's important to be very gentle with yourself. Remember, it's okay to start exactly where you are right now.

When you think back to your childhood, you'll probably remember that you used to love to run and play and couldn't wait until recess—it was natural for you to want to move your body. You may have unlearned or forgotten your inherent inclination toward being active, learning over time to focus on your aches and pains instead. Because our modern culture has made it so easy, it's likely that you've stopped incorporating activity into your daily life at all.

When you start moving again—even in small ways such as deliberately parking farther away when you go to the store and walking to your destination—you'll begin to remember how good it feels. Undoubtedly, you'll start to look forward to the times of day when you can stretch a little.

The more you move, the easier it becomes. Soon you may find yourself naturally taking up a sport that you used to appreciate and enjoy—perhaps tennis, bicycling, in-line skating, or golf. Whatever you decide to do, make sure you have fun doing it so that you'll look forward to it.

If you don't want to join a gym because of the expense, you feel uncomfortable there, or it's inconvenient, then exercise at home. I have a small, round trampoline in my closet that I pull out a few times a week and jump on. It's actually a lot of fun to put on your favorite music (particularly songs that you loved as a teenager) and dance or jump. Even if you only do a few minutes at a time, it's a wonderful place to start. Experiment with workout videos and shows. Watching TV or reading while working on a home-exercise machine or stretching may be the perfect combination for you as well.

Also, note that if you hate exercise, it may be that you aren't doing the kind you enjoy—for instance, if you like to socialize, you might want to pursue an activity that lets you do that at the same time. If you're competitive, choose something in which you compete against others or yourself (such as trying to beat your running time or the number of repetitions you do).

You'll want to set yourself up for success because each victory prepares you for the next one. Begin by setting attainable goals; then you'll begin to trust yourself, knowing that when you commit to something, you're going to keep your word and do it. So why not decide to do five jumping jacks every day when you get out of the shower, no matter what? They'll become part of your routine, just like brushing your teeth and combing your hair . . . once you get started, activity becomes part of your daily schedule.

If you experience aches and pains, remember that they won't last forever. You can break through them and reap the benefits that exercise brings. If your current weight status or health condition is such that it's difficult to do anything—even walk—check with your physician to see if you can do water exercise, which is okay for almost everyone.

I've had people tell me that they're embarrassed to go to a public pool with their bathing suit on because of their current weight. I want to encourage you to be strong, set an example for yourself and others, and go ahead and begin exercising or walking—even in public. Do this as a gift to yourself, knowing that the embarrassment is short-lived. Remember that this is a key for your long-term success.

How hard should you work out? You certainly don't want to push yourself to the point of exhaustion, but on the other hand, some of you may go to the opposite extreme of not challenging yourself at all. Find a balance and try to get in at least 30 minutes per day. Start out slowly and build up, making your goals achievable and realistic. If you've never run in your life, you may be able to do three miles the first time, but then what? How are you going to feel the next day? Are you going to want to do that again? Consistency is the key, so challenge yourself, but don't push.

On the other hand, you don't want to buy yourself a stationary bike, get on it for three minutes, decide that it's boring, and quit. Instead, it might work better for you to buy a regular, outdoor bicycle and plan a route where you can't turn back so easily. Commit to taking this path three times a week as you enjoy the fresh air and scenery. Look forward to this precious time by yourself (or with a friend) and notice how good it feels to move your body.

Associate pleasure and reward with exercise to get your subconscious mind to create the impulse to want to continue. Have the foresight to realize that if you can make this fun—even if you have to con yourself at first—it will soon become a way of life, and you will truly be permanently thinner. What a wonderful realization to have!

The methods in Part II will help you remove any blocks you have about exercising and help you look forward to it, but you should start planning your routine now. If you want to establish the natural impulse to exercise, this is what you have to program into your subconscious mind. Then, even if you have the thought that you don't feel like working out today, you'll immediately become aware of how much better you'll feel after you do—and how discouraged you'll feel if you act on that negative thought (or listen to that voice).

Before you know it, you'll start to look forward to working up a good sweat. Even aching muscles can be a positive sign (as long as you haven't overdone it). See how good it feels to have mobility in your muscles and joints, and even enjoy how refreshing a big glass of water tastes after you work out.

Here are some additional tips:

- In addition to the times when you decide to officially exercise, get into the habit of moving as much as possible throughout the day. It will make you feel better, help you sleep more soundly, and even out your energy levels.

- Stretching is very beneficial since you probably hold a lot of tension in your muscles. If you can take a Pilates or yoga class, it would be wonderful. But even if you can't fit that into your schedule right now, you can certainly begin stretching when you get out of bed in the morning or just before you go to sleep at night. If you're alone in an elevator, go for it! Take a moment to touch your toes, reach up to the ceiling, or roll your head gently from side to side.

Make it a point to stretch a little bit as often as you think of it throughout the course of the day.

- Check out the workout videos and DVDs available at your local library or video-rental store.

- Get a collection of your favorite music together on a CD or iPod and start dancing in your living room. If you prefer, you can get a small trampoline to jump on.

- Do something totally new. If you've never played tennis, for example, treat yourself to a few lessons. Find a sport or activity that you really enjoy.

- Take a local exercise class. Experiment until you discover what you find pleasurable.

- Do something "inefficiently" to get your blood moving: Take the stairs instead of the elevator, park a little farther from the store than you need to, or walk to your colleague's office or cubicle to give him or her a quick message rather than e-mailing it.

- Make a commitment to do five jumping jacks or push-ups daily—after you step out of the shower, just as the evening news is beginning, or at some other regular time. Increase the number as you become more fit.

Now that you have an idea of the foundation you can set for weight loss—and the transformation of your life—let's take a closer look at the specific food choices that can help you on your way.

CHAPTER TWO

What You Should Eat

There are some basics you need to know about a balanced, nutritious diet—beyond calories in versus calories out. You *can* lose weight by eating low-cal, unhealthy foods or by having rich meals and exercising every spare second of the day. However, the Right Weigh program is designed to help you not only achieve permanent weight loss, but also the highest level of health in mind, body, and spirit that's possible for you. What good is losing if you suffer problems due to poor nutrition, right? But with all the contradictory advice out there right now, it can be very confusing to figure out what's best.

Are You Eating the Healthiest Types of Food?

If you listen to what every expert says that you shouldn't eat, you'll go nuts! You may be familiar with these warnings:

- "Stay away from fat—it clogs your arteries" . . . yet it helps curb sugar cravings.

- "Too much sugar will do you in" . . . yet it's in everything.

- "Salt is very bad for you" . . . yet it brings flavor to the foods you eat.

- "You need protein" . . . but not too much.

- "Carbs are fattening" . . . yet they're your greatest source of energy.

No wonder you just want to give up sometimes! It's true that in excess, even the healthiest choices can potentially do harm, since you're meant to eat nutritious foods in a balanced way. By following the six steps in Part II, you'll discover how to get in touch with your body's own awareness of what it needs. For instance, as you do the exercises, you may realize that you have stomach problems whenever you drink milk or eat cheese, but you've been ignoring it because you've been told that you need calcium and these are the best sources. Making these good choices is much easier if you have a framework to guide you through all of the options out there.

The Value of Structure

You've already established that you don't want to be on a diet that causes a mentality of deprivation, but you're obviously going to have to change your eating habits. To eliminate excess hunger and create balance in your system, you'll need to start choosing healthier foods. The more you do so, the more you'll actually begin to love them.

The natural way to maintain health and an ideal weight is to trust your body, choose what it needs, and eat only when you're physically hungry. That would be a terrific plan if you were experiencing perfect balance and health right now. Chances are, however, that you're off-kilter due to years of dieting and gravitating toward unhealthy foods. Therefore, to start off, you're going to have to set some rules. Yes, this is a restriction, but it also brings much-needed structure—something that you can depend on and feel comfortable with as you rebuild trust in yourself.

Only you can make the rules. By creating this system for yourself, you won't get lost in the huge array of choices available. Think of it as adding value to your life, rather than something to rebel against. It will give you a framework to live by so that you can stop following every new fad that comes along—only to abandon the entire endeavor later on. You can begin with these preliminary steps toward your own Right Weigh program:

- Write down in your permanent-weight-loss journal three ways that you can bring yourself pleasure that have nothing to do with food. Some ideas are taking a warm bath with scented salts, listening to music you love, or taking yourself to the theater. Make a date with yourself to do at least one of those things this week.

- Establish basic meal rules for yourself. For example, only eat while sitting down at the kitchen table, no eating out of the carton, and keep the serving dishes off the table.

- Check out nutritious convenience foods at your local grocery or health-food store, and find take-out restaurants nearby that feature high-quality, fresh meals in case you have a time crunch.

- Consider ways to make your shopping and food storage more organized so that you don't run out of healthy staples and fresh produce. You might post a grocery list of veggies on your refrigerator or begin storing them in clear bags so that you don't overlook them, causing them to spoil. You can also keep an herb garden, so you can snip off herbs as you need them.

STRIKING A BALANCE

Since this is a program for the long haul, figure out what you need to do to get the results you want and still enjoy what you eat. For example, you may find that if you go to a restaurant and order a burger plain, with no bun (because it's one of the few options on the menu that isn't covered in fattening sauces) that you actually *do* feel a sense of lack. In that case, experiment with ordering the sandwich as is, but only eating a small portion of the bread.

Remember, all of the deprivation that you've subjected yourself to over the years has made your initial problem a whole lot worse. In fact, if you feel that your metabolism is so slow that you can hardly eat *anything* without gaining weight, bear in mind that it's the years of dieting that have caused this—so stop doing more of the same! Trust yourself to make healthy choices by using the tools you're learning here.

Stay in balance and don't let yourself become ravenously hungry, since that's sure to lead to a binge. Eat at regular intervals, and offset complex carbohydrates with fat and protein to slow down the amount of time it takes to burn off the calories, keeping you from experiencing excess hunger. Remember to be moderate in all of your choices and rotate your foods so that no obsessions develop.

When you eat healthfully and drink lots of pure, clean water, your natural energy level will rise, and you'll no longer need to use food as a drug. You'll feel good, so you'll find yourself wanting to move your body and be active—in fact, you'll have difficulty being sedentary anymore! If you slip up and eat things that you know are wrong for you (such as processed snacks or foods made from white flour), even if you enjoy the taste, you'll feel their negative effects. Then, like an airplane correcting its course, you'll get back on track with your healthy, supportive lifestyle.

Here are some general techniques to use as you decide what to choose and what to limit:

- Try a new, healthy food—such as a vegetable or whole grain—that you haven't had before. If you aren't sure how to prepare or store it, ask your grocer.

- The next time you have a meal, be aware of the balance of different types of food on your plate. Note whether you're eating a disproportionate amount of one category.

- Instead of buying something processed, purchase an unprocessed version. For example, rather than getting luncheon meat at the deli, buy slices of fresh turkey breast or roast your own turkey.

Now that you've started thinking about your choices, let's take a closer look at picking exactly what you'll be eating.

Foods to Choose

Although no one specific plan works for everyone, you should try to eat natural, whole, unprocessed, fresh foods with a small amount of healthy fats, and water and water-rich ingredients as much as you can. If possible, you should go organic as well.

To really keep your meal planning simple, think in terms of five categories:

1. Proteins

2. Healthy fats

3. Complex carbohydrates

4. Vegetables and fruits (although many of these are complex carbs, they have their own category)

5. Condiments (what I call the category that includes nuts, seeds, and dairy)

To keep your blood sugar steady, plan to eat three to six mini-meals a day, selecting foods from each category. When you look at your entire day, think of balancing these five groups, and do the same when you plan for the week ahead.

You may find it useful to look at your plate as if it were divided into sections, similar to a pie chart. How big a slice does the protein section of your meal cover? What about your vegetables? I choose to fill half of my plate with dark green and other veggies, and then divide the other half in two. A small sliver of that second half is for condiments such as healthy fats, sauces, dressings, nuts, and seeds. Almost a quarter of the "pie" will be whole-grain-based carbohydrates or root vegetables (such as potatoes), and the other almost-quarter will be filled with animal protein (such as fish, turkey, chicken, or other meat).

Let's take a closer look at these food categories and explore ways to help you make the best choices from each one.

PROTEINS

Whole grains and legumes are very nutritious, and if you're a vegetarian, they should be key sources of protein for you. But if you're carbohydrate sensitive, select more seafood, lean meats, and poultry instead of beans combined with dairy or grains (see Chapter 3 for more on sensitivities).

Choose animal protein that's been raised without hormones or antibiotics, and go organic whenever possible. This includes salmon, tuna, flounder (or any other kind of fish), shrimp, scallops, eggs, chicken, turkey, duck, beef, veal, and lamb. Stay away from highly processed meats such as cold cuts and hot dogs, which contain harmful additives, table salt, and sugar.

Here are some additional tips for choosing proteins:

- Check into sources of organic produce and meat. You may be able to get these products from a health-food store or food co-op. Grilling is a great option for these foods.

- Cook skinless chicken, or at least remove the skin prior to eating.

- Instead of using sweet or oily sauces, marinate your animal protein with a little bit of sesame-seed oil and Bragg Liquid Aminos (which is a wonderful salt substitute, similar to soy sauce). Sesame seeds and their oil are a good source of calcium. You won't even miss the rich, sugar-filled, nutrient-devoid sauces that you used to eat.

FATS

Another important component of good eating that will help you attain and maintain your ideal weight is incorporating healthy fats into your diet while limiting the overall amount that you consume. You're much less likely to crave the bad ones if you eat the good.

Some excellent sources of healthy fat are seeds; nuts; fish; olive, canola, and flaxseed oils (I recommend Barlean's Flax Oil); and avo-cados. Avoid margarine, fried and greasy foods, fatty or processed meat, and most vegetable oils. I also don't advocate using a lot of butter; however, a small amount on whole-grain toast with an egg is a better choice than skipping breakfast and having a candy bar later.

Here are more tips for incorporating this food group into your personal eating plan:

- Don't try to eliminate fats and sugar at the same time, since that will only work in the short run. If dairy agrees with you, enjoy some butter or cheese with your whole-grain bagel.

- If you tend to overuse fats on your salads and vegetables, flavor them instead with olive or flaxseed oil (keep refriger-ated and don't heat) mixed with apple-cider or balsamic vinegar and fresh or dried herbs, such as basil, dill, cilantro, or oregano. (Apple-cider vinegar is an especially good choice because it naturally suppresses the appetite and makes your body more alkaline. This helps balance you, since most of the foods you probably eat tend to make the body acidic.)

- Replace margarine with olive oil on bread and in cooking.

- Sauté with broth instead of vegetable oil, margarine, or butter.

- Replace fatty or processed meats with leaner cuts, such as skinless chicken, turkey, and fish.

- Incorporate avocados into your diet: Make guacamole and instead of using chips, have it with toasted pita bread or vegetable sticks. You can also use it (or sliced avocados) on sandwiches.

- Choose free-range and organic eggs and meat, which have more omega-3 fats than the regular versions.

Note: There's been a lot of research about the importance of the omega-3s in the human diet. When they're balanced with the more common omega-6 fats, they promote health in a variety of ways, including lowering the risk of heart attack and stroke. They may also reduce obesity and ease the symptoms of diabetes, as well as decrease LDL (bad) cholesterol. Researchers have found this nutrient helpful in the treatment of inflammation-related disorders such as rheumatoid arthritis, Crohn's disease, colitis, and asthma; and there have been studies on its role in reducing symptoms of bipolar disorder and depression.

CARBOHYDRATES

You may have tried to go carb-free—and even succeeded for a while and lost weight—but how long can you keep it up? Sure, avoiding carbs helps regulate blood sugar, but can you really eat that way over the long haul in real life? It's doubtful, so it's better to take a more logical approach to the two types of food in this category: simple and complex.

Sugars are simple carbohydrates, and as you know, consuming too many of these can lead to being overweight. In fact, there was a rise in obesity in this country after the public was advised to severely limit fats. This is because when your fat intake is cut or minimized, you generally won't feel satisfied, and you'll end up eating more sugar. And you'll usually consume it in the least healthy form: refined and white. Even when you read the labels of processed foods, you'll see that when fat is omitted, sugar or its substitutes are increased.

Too much of this can be deadly, putting you at greater risk for diabetes, heart failure, stroke, and, of course, obesity. Yet artificial sweeteners aren't necessarily better—in fact, many are chemicals that your body can't tolerate. They may not have calories, but it's doubtful whether they promote health and well-being. Some studies indicate that these sweeteners can actually cause weight gain because they stimulate the pancreas, causing you to want more food.

Instead of simple sugars, choose complex carbohydrates, which include grains such as brown rice, barley, whole wheat, and oats.

You can find these ingredients in many foods, including whole-grain and artichoke pasta and whole-grain or sprouted bread, tortillas, and bagels. This category also includes potatoes, sweet potatoes, beets, corn, butternut and buttercup squash, carrots, and other root vegetables, as well as fruit.

Make sure that you don't eat these foods alone (after all, a sweet potato *is* sweet). Instead, to decrease their destabilizing effect on your blood sugar, have them in combination with healthy fat and/or animal protein. Yes, that increases the calories, but it also gives you the equilibrium that your body needs and will keep you feeling satisfied longer. Think *balance.*

Here are some ways to start controlling your carb intake:

- Cut out all soft drinks, even those that are sugar-free. The chemicals in the sugar substitutes can be toxic.

- Drink plenty of fresh, pure water.

- Forget about all of those packaged "diet foods," including low-fat and low-carb bread products. Read the labels and pick ones with whole grains and minimal sweetners.

- If you're able to eat sugars, then you may be able to use organic honey, maple syrup, or date sugar with your meals.

- When you do have complex whole-grain or root-vegetable carbs, make sure to balance them by combining them with protein and healthy fat so that they break down into glucose more slowly.

- A delicious breakfast idea to help satisfy carb cravings is oatmeal. You can top it off with freshly ground golden flax-seeds, a tablespoon of almond butter, or even a couple of eggs.

- Once in a while, it's fine to prepare or buy a healthy-carb treat for yourself, such as snack bars with oats, bananas, prunes, nuts, and a dash of vanilla. If you're like I am, this may not be something that you can tolerate on a daily basis; however, if you're having an urge for sweets or need something for a long car trip, you can feel confident that these bars will satisfy you, taste good, and keep you on track.

VEGETABLES

In the vegetable department are all of the greens: collards, kale, turnip and beet greens, red and green chard, green lettuce, spring mix, spinach, and arugula. Also in this category are green and yellow squash, anise, snow peas, sprouts, broccoli, cauliflower, celery, and cabbage.

It's almost certain that you can benefit from lots of vegetables and salads, although some people can tolerate more raw foods than others. If you have digestive weaknesses, you may find it helpful to have your vegetables lightly steamed or sautéed instead of raw. This is great for fresh collards or kale: Cook them lightly in olive oil with leeks, fresh ginger and/or garlic, and a dash of sea salt.

Salads are also a delicious way to fill up, but rather than eating iceberg lettuce (which is devoid of nutrients) covered with sugar- and/or fat-laden, processed dressing, learn to enjoy delicious, healthy greens with this tasty and good-for-you salad dressing:

Mix ½ cup olive oil or Barlean's Flax Oil with ⅓ cup organic apple-cider vinegar and a teaspoon of Bragg Liquid Aminos. You can add fresh or dried garlic and herbs, if you like, using whatever you have on hand: dill, basil, oregano, parsley, cilantro, thyme, mint, and so on. Prepare a new batch once a week (it doesn't last longer than that).

Vary your veggies and try to incorporate many different colors for a variety of nutrients and flavors. You can grate beets, zucchini, red cabbage, and carrots into your salad for a delicious array of tastes (these are also great in the dressing).

If dairy isn't an offending food for you, it's okay to have as much as a tablespoon of cheese on five ounces of a spring-mix salad—if that turns your meal into something that you begin to crave above anything else! (You can use prepackaged, crumbled goat or feta cheese to make it simple.)

You can also top your veggies with some roasted pumpkin or sunflower seeds or a tablespoon of dry-roasted walnuts or pecans. If you really want some sweetness, chop one or two fresh figs for a garnish or sprinkle on a few raisins. Add some delicious, marinated animal protein, and you have a meal! And once fabulous salads become part of your routine, you'll never go back to eating bland, processed, empty foods.

FRUITS

Fruits are also wonderfully water-rich and high in vitamins, fiber, and minerals. Some people can eat them in abundance, but others— particularly those who are sensitive to sugar—need to moderate or limit their intake (see Chapter 3 for guidance on discovering sensitivities).

For a regular beverage, replace your fruit juice with plain water, or water and a splash of juice or a slice of lemon. Limit dried fruit and juice consumption and eat fiber- and water-rich fresh varieties instead.

CONDIMENTS

I place dairy, nuts, and seeds—all of which are made up of some combination of protein, carbohydrates, and fats—in a separate category called "condiments." Although they can turn a dish from boring to tasty, they need to be eaten sparingly. If consumed in excess, they often lead to weight gain (and there's strong evidence that dairy in particular contributes to illness). Also, when eaten alone, large amounts of nuts and cheese are rarely satisfying. In other words, they're likely to cause a binge, since your brain doesn't get a "feeling full" signal, despite the huge amount of calories going in.

One of my favorite condiments is Celtic Sea Salt (available at most health-food stores, or order from the Grain and Salt Society at

800-867-7258). It's dried naturally in the sun and retains all of the vital trace minerals, as you can see by its light gray color. The bits of marine life in it provide organic forms of iodine that can stay in your body much longer than that found in refined table salt. I recommend getting a salt mill and grinding it over your food—it's delicious!

Golden flaxseeds are another great way to add nutrients to your diet. Found in health-food stores, they're rich in omega-3s (healthy fat), are great for the digestive tract, and will help keep your bowel movements regular. To save time, you can grind them in your coffee grinder every few days and keep them in the refrigerator, ready to go.

You'll discover for yourself whether you can use these foods in moderation to add flavor to what you eat. If so, it's a great idea to take a mixture of raw nuts and seeds, place them on a cookie tray, lightly sprinkle them with Celtic Sea Salt, and bake on very low heat (approximately 200 degrees) for a few hours. Store in a container and sprinkle on salad or any of your other meals; this is a nutritious way to increase flavor.

Experiment with the combinations that work for you, keeping in mind what you should steer clear of . . . which may include more common foods than you think.

Foods to Avoid

Avoid sugar, sugar substitutes, additives, most vegetable oils and other unhealthy fats (such as trans fats), and table salt. Stay away from sugary sauces and processed foods as much as possible, along with any product that's mostly derived from chemicals. Read food labels and play close attention to serving sizes: Are you really only going to use a teaspoonful, which the manufacturer claims is a serving size, or will you use a tablespoon?

The next time you grocery shop, examine the nutrition information on every food that you buy on a regular basis. Familiarize yourself with the ingredients, daily values, and suggested serving sizes. In addition, these tips will help you keep making the right choices:

- Go to a health-food store and peruse the shelves for at least one new item to try, such as flaxseed oil, Bragg Liquid Aminos, toasted-sesame-seed oil, and so on.

- Consider adding animal protein to your diet to stabilize your blood-sugar levels. This will help curb carbohydrate bingeing (see Chapter 3 for more information).

- Carry around healthy snacks such as vegetable sticks (celery, carrots, cucumbers, and the like).

- Wherever you go, have some protein source with you such as meat, cheese, nuts and seeds, or yogurt—or at least make sure it's available. You can use a cooler bag for refrigeration.

SALT

Table salt is highly processed and refined. During the chemical manufacturing, all valuable magnesium and trace minerals that naturally occur in the sea are depleted.

In addition to using Celtic Sea Salt instead of commercial brands, try substituting Bragg Liquid Aminos. If you must have a salty snack at home, you can pop your own plain popcorn and top it with Bragg and nutritional yeast, a great condiment that's high in B vitamins and tastes wonderful. It satisfies that craving, and kids love it, too!

A third option, available at most grocery stores, is the combination of potassium and salt that's found in the salt section. You can also experiment with flavoring your food with dried herbs. Do use caution, however, because even a "healthy" salt will stimulate your desire for more.

DAIRY

Consuming dairy products is controversial, but your decision about whether or not to do so should be based on your individual needs. Many people will never give up their daily milk, yet those who are opposed to it have volumes of evidence supporting the fact that it's unnatural to drink milk as an adult—especially if it comes from another species!

I haven't knowingly drunk milk in years, and it feels great. On the rare occasions that I do bake a treat for myself, I use oat milk (made from just oats, and available from health-food stores) as a substitute. I can eat cheese in moderation, and even plain yogurt is something I could probably have on a very rare occasion. So you see, the avoidance rules don't *all* have to be hard and fast—just choose what works. Here are a couple of ideas to help you figure out whether this food group is for you:

- Eliminate dairy for at least seven days and see if you feel a difference in your energy level, cravings, or physical aches and pains.

- Try a cow's-milk substitute such as rice, soy, almond, or oat milk.

SOY

Soy, like dairy, is a food that some people do well with, and others need to avoid. There's a lot of literature available about its cancer-fighting and cholesterol-lowering properties, but the best way to know if it's good for you is to keep track of how you feel when you eat it. Some people have obvious negative reactions (such as fatigue or headaches), while others find it to be an excellent vegetarian source of protein.

If you do choose to eat these products, make sure to read the labels, because a lot of the commercial soy sauces are filled with additives such as corn syrup and caramel color. Select a natural, good-quality product that's brewed in wooden kegs for months and is only made with water, soybeans, and sea salt. Many high-quality options (such as tamari and the product labelled "shoyu") have been fermented, which enhances their enzyme content, making the food more easily assimilated and digested.

Tofu itself has a bland taste, but it's extremely versatile in picking up the flavors of whatever it's cooked with. Try marinating it or tempeh in sugar-free dressings such as tahini (crushed sesame-seed paste) and miso (a fermented-soy product) to give them flavor. You can then broil, bake, or sauté them with vegetables.

You've learned a lot so far, but don't worry—a healthy eating plan doesn't have to be complicated.

Planning Ahead—It Really Can Be Easy!

Once you've started making nutritious choices, just adapt them as the circumstances require. If you're hosting guests who aren't eating the way you do, you can easily serve chicken and just take the skin off of your own piece, helping yourself to a generous portion of vegetables to ensure that you really enjoy your meal.

If you're cooking steak on the grill, marinate it in a tasty, homemade, sugar-free sauce; have yours with a big, nutritious salad. And when you give your children a treat, make sure that you aren't hungry. If you are, have a healthy snack before serving them. In fact, why not offer them the nutritious choice first?

When you're on the road, you can take food with you in a plastic container with an ice pack. If you're pressed for time, it only takes a moment to throw a bag of salad into a container, put a little of your homemade dressing on top, and add a package of tuna for protein. Once you get in the habit of taking meals along, you'll realize that you're actually saving time and money. You'll be able to enjoy delicious, healthy food without the time-consuming task of looking—and paying—for such options when you're out.

Being prepared is a necessary component in your strategy for success. I could never have been so successful over the last 18 years if I hadn't planned ahead. If you do forget to bring your own supplies, however, there's no need to panic. Just determine what your body needs in the moment, and make the best possible choices from what's available at the time.

WHAT TO EAT WHEN YOU'RE OUT

You don't have to be neurotic about your healthy new lifestyle. Even if you're forced to eat out a lot of the time, it's much easier to make good choices today than it was in the past. Even fast-food chains offer better options than they used to, such as plain baked potatoes and salad bars.

When you're at a party or restaurant, just relax and make the best selection that you can. Eat half of the food in front of you and take the rest home for another meal or give it to someone else. If possible, get up and leave the table before dessert is served. Don't linger; instead, get involved in another activity.

Most restaurants have olive oil and vinegar available, which you can use sparingly as a dressing. You can order a broiled fish or chicken sandwich and take off the bread (or only eat half of it). Salmon with lemon and butter is another wonderful choice. Yes, the butter is high in fat and calories, but in moderation, it will satisfy you and won't stimulate sugar cravings the way that rich, creamy preparations could (so it's the lesser evil compared with Alfredo or wine sauces).

Choosing to have all of your food plain (no butter, salt, or the like) may be the healthiest decision, but if you aren't enjoying your food, you'll probably just binge later. When you plan your strategy, keep reminding yourself that this isn't a short-term approach. You're reconditioning your brain to develop new habits. Thin people enjoy food, and you can, too—but you do need to change your perceptions and taste. Simply decide that you're worth it, turn in the direction of your goal, and never look back.

But what if you just can't stop thinking about cookies . . . or bread? There may be more at work than just a casual desire for those foods, and the next chapter will help you get to the bottom of it.

CHAPTER THREE

Food Cravings and Addictions

It would be so easy to turn this into just another diet book and make up a plan for you. But those regimens don't work because they create a psychologically temporary situation. The moment you go on one, you're waiting for the second when you can quit! The Right Weigh program, on the other hand, permanently alters the way in which you think about food. And when your thoughts change, your behavior will as well. You'll stay motivated to stick with a sensible plan without feeling deprived and restricted.

So you know that you need to burn more calories than you consume, and you're aware of great healthy food options . . . but why is it so difficult sometimes to make the right choices? Much of the bingeing you do is simply your attempt to feel better and put your body in balance. Unfortunately, many times you're inadvertently causing the opposite effect: Instead of creating health, your habits are pushing you toward fatigue, illness, depression, and being overweight. With the information in this chapter, you'll be able to not only lose your excess weight, but also live your life filled with high energy and the best of health. I speak from experience. . . .

My Story of Sugar Addiction

Eliminating sugar from my life in 1986 was the best thing I ever did for myself. I want to share with you that this possibility not only exists, but that it can completely set you free and make worries about your weight a thing of the past.

Because my father was diabetic and I always loved sugar as a child, I'm sure that I inherited the genes that caused me to have a preexisting impulse toward sweet foods. Before I began eating the way I do now, I had very strong cravings, and I think that a lot of them were due to an imbalance in my metabolism caused by undiagnosed hypoglycemia.

When I first started feeling sick and tired all the time, I began to associate extreme pain with the foods I used to love. Every time I looked at cake or cookies, I pictured myself feeling exhausted for days. I used the sensation and the internal picture of being sick to my benefit and associated it with the offending dishes (whether or not they were actually causing my illness).

I imagined that sugar, alcohol, and caffeine could lead me to even greater health problems, such as diabetes and all of the complications associated with it (blindness, loss of a limb, and so on). I wanted to create enough momentum in my own being to stay away from sugar, no matter what environment I was in.

When I looked at salads and vegetables, however, I imagined that they held the nutrients that were going to bring my health back and sustain me. After a few failed attempts at achieving wellness through vegetarianism, I succumbed to the fact that I needed animal protein. I made sure to eat meat (beef, chicken, or fish) regularly throughout the day, and I incorporated healthy fats into my diet, which made my food taste great.

This transformation wasn't about suffering. I decided to give myself the gift of health and honor the body that God had blessed me with. If you've ever been sick, you can relate to the gratitude I felt to be given a second chance.

As it turned out, the low heart rate and irregular heartbeat that had landed me in the hospital, where I received a pacemaker at the age of 26, may have been caused by an infection that went to my heart—not just poor eating and exercise habits. When I learned this, I was tempted to think that my food choices weren't really as important as I'd previously assumed, since it was probably my low heart rate that had caused the overwhelming fatigue.

Although no doctor confirmed for me that my diet needed to be restricted, my inner wisdom told me otherwise. I had a deep inner knowing that I was finally free from my attachment to unhealthy eating habits, and that going back to eating sugar moderately would be traveling down a road to suffering. I knew that I'd been addicted and obsessed—and I didn't want to go back there.

Identifying Problem Areas

Do certain foods cause *you* to crave others? For example, how do you feel when you eat eggs for breakfast versus oatmeal? Do you feel better when you have toast or juice with your eggs, or do you notice repeatedly that you feel better when you just have them plain? If you buy a container of yogurt, do you obsess about it until it's gone (a sign that you have an imbalance), or can you take it or leave it (in which case, it's more likely to be a healthy choice for you)?

When you crave things, it's often because of the types of foods you've been eating. You may think that you simply want, say, a big submarine sandwich piled high with processed, fatty meat for lunch, but what's really happening is that the food you ate for breakfast—or that fact that you skipped the morning meal—is the cause of your desire.

Often, these patterns aren't totally obvious. Are you crazy for bananas because you need potassium, or is it just a sugar imbalance? What happens when you eat different things—do the desires disappear? A great way to discover whether you have a sensitivity, or even a food addiction, is by tracking what you eat in a specific way.

USING A FOOD DIARY

Figuring out which foods truly do support you can be of immeasurable help, particularly if you're unsure as to whether certain ingredients are good for you or harmful. Your food diary can be a small notepad or spiral notebook that you carry around with you wherever you go, or it can be part of your permanent-weight-loss journal. Set up your notes like the example on the following page:

Date	Time of Day	Rate Feeling, 1–10	Food I Desire	Food I Eat	Feeling Immediately Following, 1–10	One Hour Later	Three Hours Later	Next Day

FOOD DIARY

To rate your feelings, use this scale:

Emotional and Physical Scale, 1–10
   1: Depressed, tired, sad, and awful
   5: Neutral
  10: Top of the world, exuberant, peaceful, and calm

As you can see, you should log not only what you eat and when, but what your feelings are before, during, and after choosing particular foods. Are you attracted to certain dishes when you're experiencing specific emotions? Take notes about how you feel one hour after you eat, three hours later, and even the next day.

Over the course of several days or weeks, you'll probably start to see patterns. Notice what you ate earlier on days when you feel obsessed with having something you really shouldn't eat. Pay attention to what you consumed at times when you felt totally satisfied, and food didn't enter your mind until you were physically hungry.

I recommend that you use this diary for at least four days, but preferably for a couple of weeks. If you find evidence that something might be causing you to yearn for foods you'd like to avoid—or even that you may have an addiction to something—don't despair. As you'll learn, you can free yourself from these desires and possibly even reintroduce a food back into your diet at a later date.

IF YOU HAVE MORE THAN ONE PROBLEM FOOD

If using your food diary reveals that you probably have more than one problem food, start changing your habits slowly. You may see articles that tell you to eliminate all fruit, white flour, and carbohydrates. While this can be helpful (especially initially) because it helps purge all possible offenders from your body and frees you from the endless cycle of addiction, this approach also presents the risk of overwhelming you—and might even cause you to fail. Instead, cut out the obvious first. For example, if carbohydrates are a problem, just eliminate sugar in its most concentrated and blatant forms.

For at least ten days, completely avoid the food that you think causes you the most trouble: cravings, the impulse to eat a very large portion, physical problems such as headaches, and so on. After ten days, that trigger will have cleared itself from your system and you'll have a better sense of whether the other things you're eating are causing you problems or if this was the culprit. Also, eliminating that first item may dramatically reduce your cravings for other foods, making it easier for you to cut them out.

Controlling Cravings

This is the point where you can refine the basic rules you made in Chapter 2. You may still think that you want the freedom to make any food choice. However, if you live that way, you're likely to make decisions that are harmful, particularly when you're under stress. When you've established boundaries such as: "I don't drink caffeine or eat sugar," and this is a rule you're deeply committed to for the greater good of your life, then you'll be motivated to automatically find new ways to cope with stress, such as regularly exercising and eating healthy foods that you really enjoy so that you don't have a sense of lack.

If you don't have structure, you're likely to bounce back and forth between two extremes. There will be periods when you're on a diet and doing very well. But then what happens? You'll go from total restriction to absolute chaos. You *need* rules—not short-term ones such as when you're on a diet, but guidelines that will help you live and eat according to principles that will ultimately assist you in having the life you desire.

MONITOR YOUR MEALS

To help figure out this specific information to control your cravings, use your food diary to discover how often you need to eat to keep your blood sugar stabilized. How long can you go before your stomach is growling, you have a headache, or you feel light-headed or irritable? These are all signs that you need something in your belly.

When you go too long without food, your blood-sugar levels drop and your body craves a quick fix—usually sugar, white flour, saturated fat, or a combination of all three—which it knows will stop that famished feeling immediately. Yes, consuming these will satiate you, but they aren't the best choices. What's more, they'll actually cause you to want more of them. This puts you on a roller coaster of overeating, causing your blood sugar to dive, and then you'll just consume these processed ingredients again.

If you've been letting the clock dictate mealtimes, you need to get in the habit of eating when you're physically hungry; then only have the amount you need to satisfy your body, and no more. Again, three to six minimeals (or a combination of meals and snacks) each day is better than being hungry for extended stretches.

If you do slip up one day and overindulge in a particular food that you're trying to limit, rather than panic, you can simply tip the scale in the other direction the next day. The secret to success is to enjoy it, not feel guilty, and then get right back to your healthy choices as soon as possible.

For example, you may find yourself at a gathering where the only option is pizza. Eat it if necessary, but balance that by making sure that you select water or seltzer as a beverage. Enjoy the slice to the fullest, yet even as you savor the taste (as well as the socializing), maintain an awareness of the high salt and fat intake. Don't block it out. This will discourage any fantasizing about eating such food on a regular basis. If you get bloated or feel uncomfortable after you eat, pay attention to that feeling—it's vital feedback from your body.

Then, later on that day or the next, have some raw vegetables, particularly lettuce and celery, which will help your body get back in balance so that you don't find yourself on a carbohydrate binge. Sauté or steam some broccoli as soon as you can, and eat that to get back into harmony. Make sure to log the entire experience in your food diary.

Let's take a closer look at a few common triggers for cravings, such as that pizza, and then some general tips to help you stay on track.

CARBOHYDRATES

When your health is compromised, you may tend to have more cravings in terms of sweeteners, caffeine, refined carbohydrates, and alcohol. Often, you'll end up self-medicating with these substances.

If you simply must have carbs but aren't satiated when you do, you may be sensitive to them. Eating a high-carb diet regularly will create an imbalance in your system because you'll always need more and feel hungry, even though your body is stuffed with food. It's like a hunger in your brain. You're not getting the nutrients your body needs, despite the fact that you may be eating salad, vegetables, rice, and beans. Here are a couple of possible solutions:

- Put meat into the mix on a regular basis. This will get your body back in balance and foster health, especially when you eat it in combination with smaller portions of carbs (preferably the complex ones). Your meals should focus more on vegetables and protein and less on rice or pasta.

- Incorporate the healthy fat your body needs to move back into balance. A craving for potato chips or chocolate could simply be a sign that your body needs additional dietary fat. I found that when I increased my intake of flaxseeds, olive and flaxseed oil, avocados, and salt-free nuts, a lot of my desires for processed foods subsided.

DAIRY

Many people have a strong connection to dairy—especially milk. But when you feel so attached to having something, you may begin to wonder: *Is there an addiction at play here that may not be so healthy after all?* The dairy association and similar advocates will tell you that you need milk to make your bones grow. In fact, you *do* need calcium and protein—but there are other sources, such as dark leafy greens and sesame seeds.

Many experts believe that this food group contributes to or even causes arthritis, food allergies, obesity, a weakened immune system, and much more. How do you feel when you consume it? You might say, "I feel great—it energizes me." Well, really pay attention: Is it a type of "high" that you get, only to crash later and want more? If so, that sounds like addiction.

I speak from experience here: I loved the taste of milk, and when I first stopped eating ice cream, it was such a pleasure to top my foods with plain yogurt as an alternative. I even used it as a substitute for sour cream (which was a definite no-no for me). However, I soon had to come to terms with the fact that even plain yogurt—with no extra sugars or additives, coming straight from the health-food store—caused me to have cravings. I don't like the feeling of being obsessed with a certain item, or even food in general, so I stopped eating it.

Use your food diary to determine your dietary strengths and weaknesses. After a week or two, you'll have a clearer idea of what path you should take—and please don't hesitate to consult a nutritionist to make sure that you still get enough calcium if you decide to cut back here.

SUPPLEMENTS

The same process of inquiry should be applied to the supplements you're taking. You can read all about the benefits of magnesium, for example, or the importance of doing a liver cleanse, but only your own body can tell you if they're truly what you need right now.

When you're taking a supplement for overall health, you often might not be aware of its effect on you at all—you just know that it's good for you. However, there may be situations where one of these products is actually causing you to feel fatigue or cravings. If you suspect that this is the case, using your food diary to record your emotions and physical state both when you take the supplement and when you eliminate it for a few days can be very helpful.

WHEN IN DOUBT

Here are some general tips for filling yourself up in a healthy way, which will help you stave off all sorts of cravings:

- Consider using fiber supplements to help your digestive tract and fill you up. AIM Natural Health makes an excellent fiber powder that I highly recommend. It doesn't taste good, but in my experience it stabilizes blood sugar and eliminates cravings. It's also available in capsule form.

- If you feel sluggish or bloated, try drinking the juice of one whole lemon and a teaspoon of olive oil in a cup of hot water daily for one or two weeks upon arising.

- Try a tablespoon of Organic Raw Apple Cider Vinegar (available at health-food stores) or lemon juice in a glass of water before every meal. This can help with cravings and assist you in eating less.

- Prepare a broth of boiled vegetables (roots and greens, perhaps with ginger, garlic, and onion); you can freeze some of it to use later. Sip this throughout the day. It will give you vitamins and minerals and help fill you up, too. Take some with you in an insulated container when you go out. (Health-food stores have wonderful organic broths, without all the salt and additives, to use as soup bases.)

- Slice fresh ginger and boil it in water to make tea. This is a wonderful beverage that will cleanse your system and help you stay healthy. Ginger is excellent for the immune system and digestive tract.

- If you usually enjoy a food that isn't very fresh, find a substitute: freshly baked, whole-grain bread instead of store-bought; fresh fish instead of frozen; and so on.

- Prepare nutritious staples once a week. Make your own salad dressing, vegetable soup, or rice, and broil or bake marinated chicken or salmon to pull out when you don't have time to cook.

- Keep mixed field greens on hand; if you're in a hurry, you can simply dress and eat them.

- Try a moderate amount of the food you're craving. For instance, you may be able to get away with feeding your sweet tooth with homemade cookies, made without sugar and sweetened only with raisins or fresh or dried fruit.

Can your body tolerate a small amount of a given food without slipping over the edge? Only you can determine your options. With some experimentation, guided by your deep inner wisdom and what you've discovered by using your food diary, you'll get clear about what you can get away with and what's absolutely *not* an option . . . perhaps because you're addicted.

"No Longer an Option"—Food Addiction

If you find yourself simply unable to control your intake of a certain ingredient—regardless of what tricks you use—then you're very likely addicted to it. I strongly recommend that you put such foods in a "no longer an option" category. This means that eating sugar, for example, is one of the behaviors you simply don't engage in, just as you would never rob a bank because you were financially stressed, or punch someone because you were angry.

You might say, "Well, of course I would never do *those* things because of the consequences and because I know it's not right." Ask yourself why it's right to hurt yourself so deeply through your food choices. Why is it okay to consistently engage in behavior that's causing you so much physical and emotional pain?

Once you make this inner connection, it becomes easy to recognize and accept that sugar, to continue with that example, isn't your friend. With love and compassion for yourself (not with a whip), make a commitment to no longer choose to eat it. Affirm to yourself that you're willing to find new, healthy sources of pleasure and ways to reduce stress that nourish you on every level of your being.

FACING THE PROBLEM

You may have trouble believing that you actually have an addiction. After all, sugar and white flour are in practically everything, and almost everybody eats them. Start to track your own personal experience when you eat dishes high in whatever your problem ingredient may be. You can certainly find many books that include information on the perils of different diets, but it's important for you to discover for yourself what impact these foods are having on your life.

For the next month, keep a chart in your food diary of your cravings, what you eat, and how you feel. Look back over the last year and think about how you've struggled with uncontrollable desire and its consequences. Once your addiction becomes apparent to you, you'll be motivated to take control of your life, stop the yo-yo dieting, and kick this once and for all.

Your spouse, your kids, and your best friend may be able to eat certain things with no reaction, while the same items make you experience intense cravings. Once you accept yourself, the fact that someone else can eat that food becomes irrelevant. This is similar to the way that it's pointless for an alcoholic to ask, "Why can Mary have a glass of wine with dinner, and I can't?" A dry alcoholic (one who's chosen to be sober) knows and accepts his fate and appreciates his life sober. That's because he knows the alternative: The memory of the pain inflicted by the booze is strong enough that he's sure to never re-create it.

Similarly, when you realize what's at play, it's important for you to admit that you can't master it. You've tried, and it's evident that you can't. You therefore have a choice: Either the addiction controls you, wreaking havoc on your health, moods, energy level, and life in general; or you make a commitment to do whatever it takes to free yourself so that you can reach your highest potential.

If you don't acknowledge and accept this fact, then when you feel weak or are having moments of stress, you'll convince yourself that you can cheat and handle the foods that are poisonous to your system. So take a serious look at what you're consuming on a regular basis and how it's affecting your mental and physical health. If you're dealing with a food addiction, then it may be impossible to continue your intake without feeling the negative effects.

FREEDOM FROM ADDICTIVE FOODS

If you do choose to eat addictive foods (such as sugar, salty or oily things, dairy, and so on), even in moderation, realize that it's very likely that you're making the choice to continue to have cravings that you're going to have to fight against. How strong these impulses will be depends on your genetics, health condition, body type, and other factors such as stress. You may be very successful at blocking out or controlling the desire at certain times, but it's important for you to be aware that these feelings are likely if the offending ingredients are still in your system.

The other choice, as I mentioned, is eliminating the addictive substance completely. Even though this may seem like the more difficult choice, it's actually the easier road for many people. Once you stop eating a certain category of food, you no longer crave it. Sure, once in a while you may see or smell it and feel some desire. But normally, the need is much milder than ever before and very manageable.

If you do choose to eliminate addictive foods, use the exercises in Step 5 (page 135) to change your perceptions of pleasure and pain. Even with a challenging weakness, such as chocolate, you can transform your inner reactions by practicing so that the problem food becomes disgusting to you.

Even in your everyday, waking state, you can imagine that this item is covered in mud, or think of some other image that makes it repulsive to you. This is the opposite of fantasizing. When you use fantasy, you imagine how wonderful something will be: the taste, smell, and texture—and even the good feelings associated with it. Although these emotions may be nothing more than a subconscious response to a television commercial, for example, that had a good song playing in the background or some beautiful people walking around half naked, the positive aura that's evoked seems so real and tangible that it leads to desire.

What that fantasy blocks out, however, is how bad you'll actually feel if you choose to indulge in the enticing dish. Even if you do have positive feelings during the experience, they'll be very short-lived . . . and followed by suffering.

It's important to retrain yourself to associate the addictive food with pain, because in those moments of indulgence, it's easy to forget the suffering it causes you after the initial pleasure is over. Remember that you hate being fat, and it's awful to be out of control, anticipating the next "fix." This is what you need to feel when you're tempted to eat the problematic ingredient if you're going to keep yourself from wanting it.

I didn't have to imagine anything so graphic as bugs in my food to turn me off to the foods I was addicted to. All I had to do was tune in to those miserable feelings of being overweight (and being sick and tired all the time), and I could easily say no, because I knew what was perpetuating those conditions within me. And even though I was still feeling bad for a period of time after I changed my habits, I just knew that if I continued to avoid sugar and eat healthy foods, I would heal. That was where my faith came in.

The other side of the coin is that when you're selling yourself on the idea of letting go of your addiction, it's important to also use the benefits approach and really look forward to what this will do to improve the quality of your life. Let your natural inclination toward pleasure (and away from pain) work in your favor.

When I eliminated sugar, caffeine, and alcohol from my diet, I started to focus on all of the positive aspects of living without these substances. My first reward was the vast improvement in my health, and my energy and concentration soared. I also liked the freedom of not having a scale in my house and fitting into all of my "skinny" clothes.

Abstaining from addictive foods doesn't mean that you can't

socialize or enjoy what you eat to the fullest. When you free yourself from obsession, not only do you give yourself the gift of freedom, you open space in your life for something new and wonderful to come in. What a relief to be finished with the neuroses about dieting and weight that simply drained your energy!

Trust in the Process

When you first break free of food addiction, you may not see instant results in terms of your weight or your health, but you must trust that you'll achieve your outcome if you keep heading in the right direction. It's a natural law that engaging in healthy behaviors (eating well, exercising, getting enough sleep, and practicing deep relaxation or meditation regularly) will lead to a better state of well-being than not doing so. Remain very conscious of what the likely alternative will be if you continue in the old way.

Even if your results aren't dramatic initially, eating smaller portions of healthier foods increases the likelihood of more positive developments over the long run. Sure, you could lose ten pounds the first month or see an instant burst in your energy level. But over the long term, you must be realistic and expect that you'll hit plateaus—times when choosing the "right" behaviors doesn't budge the numbers on the scale.

Perhaps you're exercising every day but you still feel tired. If this is the case, be aware of the likelihood of negative self-talk creeping in: "This doesn't work," "I knew it," "Why should I bother with this?" "I might as well enjoy my life," and so on. These are sabotaging voices, and you'll soon know what to do with them (use the exercises in Steps 4 and 5 to extinguish them immediately, or call a supportive person who can help you get past those feelings).

Always keep the story of the tortoise and the hare in mind: Slow and steady wins the race. If you just keep going in the right direction—even if it seems like you aren't making any progress at all—you *will* arrive at your destination. Whenever you're tempted to turn back, remember how far you've come; where you're going; and your commitment to yourself, your life, and your faith.

Reintroducing Foods

Bear in mind that any decision to completely eliminate a food is reversible. Although I've never gone back to eating dishes with an obviously high-sugar content (such as ice cream, store-bought cake, or cookies), which I eliminated from my diet years ago, I *have* been able to reintroduce low-sugar foods in moderation (such as bread, mayonnaise, and ketchup).

Your body's needs and ability to tolerate certain foods fluctuate, so don't think in black or white: "I want it all the time" or "I'll never get to have it." That's the voice of deprivation. Your tastes will change and your choices will increase over time.

For example, if you eliminate cheese entirely, try eating cheese again in three months. Maybe start with goat cheese this time, which is easier for many people to tolerate, and see how your body responds. As you get healthier, you can start to incorporate a greater variety into your diet. Sometimes the things that used to disagree with you can be added back in with moderation.

Take out your permanent-weight-loss journal and create some more rules for yourself (or modify the ones you've already established). Make three lists, using the following headings:

- Foods I Choose to Eat
- Foods That Are Okay in Moderation
- Foods That Are No Longer an Option

Using what you've learned in the first part of this book, fill in as much information as you can . . . and get ready to permanently transform your weight and your life with the exercises in Part II.

THE SIX-STEP PROGRAM

CHAPTER FOUR

An Overview of the 40-Day Plan

All the knowledge you've acquired about the importance of healthy, nutritious, water-rich, unprocessed food and the necessity of physical activity is useless without an understanding of how your subconscious mind is getting in the way of following through on your conscious desires. No matter how much you've wished that you could be thin and healthy and moderate in your eating, if you've held the picture of yourself as overweight and unhealthy as the dominant thought in your mind, you've been steadily moving toward the results that you don't want. Instead of continuing to go down this path, you can reverse your thinking about yourself in order to achieve the outcome you desire.

It's natural at times to feel a sense of inner conflict as you begin the process of reprogramming your mind—that is, by making use of the exercises in this section of the book and working with (instead of against) the pleasure-pain principle you'll learn about. However, this program will instill new habits and beliefs, and you'll find it increasingly natural to exercise instead of remaining sedentary, and to eat nutritiously instead of unhealthfully.

Why 40 Days?

You should stay on each of the six steps for at least one week before moving on to the next, so it will take about 40 days to work through all of them. You see, studies show that it takes at least 40 days to break a habit and create new thought patterns in the brain, and thus new automatic behaviors. Even though it will take you longer than this to get down to the weight where you feel comfortable and good about yourself, once you change the basic components, your success is certain.

Note that this plan calls for you to devote at least 30 minutes every day to the exercises in the following chapters—this time commitment is one of the greatest gifts you can give yourself. Choose to do them in a place where you won't be disturbed, and schedule it into your planner. You're worth it. Resist any temptation to talk yourself out of following through.

After the 40 days, taking time to do the exercises will be a habit. Continue to use the ones you've most benefited from, or if you feel that you need the structure, you can certainly begin the program again and use it until you achieve your ideal weight—and even longer.

How to Work the Six Steps

In the following steps, you'll find exercises that correspond to each of the six steps in the 40-day Right Weigh plan; every step has three to six tasks within it. It's best to read through the entire step and practice each exercise at least once. Then, consider which ones resonate with you most deeply and pick those that you want to implement for the rest of the week.

I'd like you to try each activity, but you can just discard the ones that don't work for you (with the exception of certain exercises from Step 1 that you'll be asked to do every day for the entire duration of the program). In addition, I want you to notice the visual cues in your environment that trigger your eating behaviors, and then the reminders that you'll create to reinforce your vision, which you'll learn about in Exercise 5.

It's perfectly fine to combine two or more of the exercises. In fact, many of my clients find it helpful to begin their program for the day by starting with Exercise 7: Grounding or Exercise 22: Personal Affirmative Prayer (or at least some version of them). And although it's more time-consuming, it's also a great idea to continue to regularly work with all of your chosen activities for the week.

All the pieces of the program build on each other, so it's important to read through—and do—them in order. Later on, after you've gone through the program once, you can repeat any piece of it for as long as you like. Also, if there's a certain exercise in Step 3, for example, that really helps you, but you've moved on to another step, simply continue with that activity in addition to your current work. In other words, you can keep doing things that help, but don't jump ahead.

If it seems as if I'm giving you a lot of exercises, remember that your old programming has been in your brain for a long time. For the best chance of success, you need to flood your subconscious mind with positive suggestions to help replace the old, worn-out, negative self-talk, and each exercise offers you a unique way to begin to break down the programming that has led you to unproductive habits.

WHEN SHOULD YOU DO THE EXERCISES?

Right now, 30 minutes a day may sound like a lot, and you might feel as if you don't have that kind of time, especially with all of your other commitments. As I assured you, once you give yourself the gift of this time, you'll wonder how you ever got along without it.

If your life is very busy, try doing the exercises early in the morning or at night before you go to sleep. These are times of day when your subconscious is more open, and you can more easily slip into deeper levels of awareness. If you find yourself falling asleep during the exercise, try sitting up instead of lying down.

You may also want to try lunchtime or just after a busy workday, or you can experiment if you don't naturally gravitate to one time in particular. Notice the difference when you do the exercises at dawn versus midday and find what works best for you. The most important thing is simply to start so that you can get a taste of their incredible benefit.

At this point in my life, I often do these exercises for one hour sometime between 2 and 5 A.M. If this works for you, you may find yourself waking up naturally to practice. I know that I find this time of the night to be incredibly peaceful, which adds a sublime quality to the experience. I can feel my connection to my deeper self blossoming, and I know that my requests are being answered. It's so much easier to focus inward without the distractions of the physical world.

Regardless of when you perform the activities in the following chapters—they'll begin to have a tangible effect on your outer life. You'll start to realize that there's a deeper place within you, beyond the daily turmoil. It doesn't mean that you won't get caught up in your day-to-day life and the world around you, but you'll now have the possibility of responding from a more centered place.

For the longest time, I was so concerned with losing sleep. It was—and still is—so important to me, and I know that sleep is a necessary component for health. Yet when I started to shorten my dreamtime by getting up early to meditate, I actually felt better during the day since I was being rejuvenated on a much deeper level. Also, even though I loved getting lots of rest, I didn't realize how much of it had been disturbed by nightmares or waking up. Although I was getting a little less sleep, it was of a better quality: It felt deeper and calmer, and the nightmares miraculously stopped (after 30 years of having them). Also, when I chose to do my meditation in the daytime, I inevitably got caught up in the many demands of the day, and either didn't do it or had difficulty focusing.

I was motivated to make this time an absolute priority by reminding myself that I was at the end of the road and had already tried every possible alternative. Don't you sometimes feel that way, too? Haven't you been on enough diets? Is the new one that comes out next year really going to be that different? And is it worth living your life with your health compromised or having to take medications that inevitably have side effects? Haven't you experienced enough pain already?

Make the time. You'll be glad you did.

Enlist the Support of a Friend

It's a wonderful plan to have a buddy travel this path with you. Find a partner who wants to achieve permanent weight loss as much as you do and is willing to make the journey. You can take turns guiding each other through the exercises (instead of recording them) or just being there for support. This person can also be helpful in gently bringing you back on course when you inadvertently slip—pulling you back from negative thinking and the voices that sabotage you. Together you can learn to change the way you relate to yourselves and your issues around food.

If you have more than one friend who'd like to do the Right Weigh program, you may even want to start a support group so you can encourage each other as you move toward a healthier life and freedom from addiction. This is an inward journey, yet it's extremely helpful to have allies along the way to help you through any rough spots.

If you're like most people, you started out by following an external route, seeking answers out in the world. One way you may have done so is by getting therapy or turning to close friends for answers and guidance. Counseling can be extremely helpful because it provides a nonjudgmental healing environment, yet it's also important to be aware of its possible limitations. If your problems are being addressed only at the conscious level, you can end up constantly regurgitating your old beliefs and reliving your past experiences . . . and staying stuck in them.

Naturally, therapists (and friends who aren't taking the journey with you) can be very supportive and loving, but unfortunately, they're just as likely to buy into your stories as you are. In order to be free, you need to move past the old images, memories, and limited realities, no matter how much of an impact they may have had on you. Yes, the incidents may have shaped you—it's tragic that some of us have grown up in environments that were hurtful physically or emotionally—but now these very experiences can serve to teach you about your own inner strength, wisdom, compassion, and ability to forgive.

It can be very helpful to become aware of the tendency for people who care about you to buy into your story and support you from the very role that you're trying to break free of, such as the victim or abuser. A woman who's tired of identifying herself as a bulimic, angry at her parents, and always struggling because she overeats might not be able to actually stop the pattern until she lets go of her self-image as "the angry bulimic who's a victim of her parents' neglect." Unless the people she's seeking help from are seeing beyond her life story to a higher perception than she can imagine, it's unlikely that they'll be able to help her break free.

The Right Weigh approach is designed to empower you to reject limiting stories about yourself and see, feel, and know the truth of who you really are: a beautiful, innocent, loving child of God. If you can, find a friend who's willing to open her perception and see herself (and you) in this way, too.

What to Do If You Feel Resistant

There may be a part of you that's hesitant to give up old beliefs and habits easily after the years you've spent struggling with them. And at times, you may find yourself reluctant to practice the exercises or be skeptical of their value. I encourage you to go past that feeling and just do them. Your commitment is only for 40 days, and it will all be so much easier after that!

As you read through the following tools and techniques, you might wonder how anything so simple could have any real impact on the problems you've carried around for years. As basic as they seem, when these exercises are performed regularly, they can completely transform your life. Don't let their simplicity fool you.

You might wonder, *If it's so easy, then why did I struggle for so long?* Be kind to yourself. You won't always know why you had periods in your life that were extremely painful, or times when you felt completely stuck. That shouldn't deter you from coming out of the rut when you're guided to do so and have the assistance you need.

This book is your guide, but it will only work if you use the tools. Just reading it will make a minimal impact on your life, but if you go through it and realize, *That makes sense, so I'm going to give it a try*— and then follow through—you'll experience tremendous gains. At the very least, if you aren't ready to commit to the entire program, I challenge you to just attempt one of the exercises every day for 40 days and see if it doesn't make a difference in your beliefs, feelings, and behaviors. Then ask yourself, *What might happen if I follow through with the entire program?*

WHAT IF THE PLAN ISN'T WORKING?

Please don't judge your results prematurely—after all, you didn't gain all your excess pounds in a week. Give yourself the gift of time, no matter how desperate you may feel. It's so important that you commit to the entire 40-day, six-step plan. Do it for yourself, be patient, and trust that you'll be able to manifest your vision of a healthy, fit body at an ideal weight. Keep your eye on the goal.

Practicing the exercises regularly will help you develop the trust and patience that you require, because the more you practice each lesson, the more powerful it becomes. You'll actually begin to experience a shift in your internal programming. In the same way that you build a set of muscles by using them, you'll increase your ability to communicate internally the more you do so. Soon you'll be able to maintain your strong connection to your inner Source of guidance, wisdom, patience, and perseverance, even in the face of chaos all around you. From this center, you'll be better equipped to respond to your outer circumstances. You'll start to become aware of more choices, especially those that will ultimately lead to the results you want for yourself.

Getting Started

Get out your permanent-weight-loss journal, a package of 3" x 5" or 4" x 6" index cards, a tape recorder, and a dozen blank tapes with labels, all of which I mentioned in Chapter 1.

Remember, every step has particular exercises for you to do over the course of that week. However, there are a few short but powerful ones you'll begin doing while working on a certain step and then continue for the duration of the program. For example, the first one is imagining your vision, which you'll create in Step 1. So each day you'll reread the index card on which you've written your vision and take a moment to actually *imagine* your desired outcome, giving yourself credit for successes and taking note of any failures.

Also, every day throughout the program, take a few moments here and there to follow through with Exercise 5: Create Visual Cues to Reinforce New Beliefs. Part of this task includes declaring your new behaviors and goals to yourself as you go through the day (when you're in the shower, while you're driving, or waiting in line). Stay aware of the visual cues in your environment.

Throughout the course of the 40 days, I'd like you to reread the chapter for the week as you work the step. The rationale provided within those pages will help you stay motivated. So, for example, on the first day of Step 1, you'll read Chapter 5 and the exercises for that step. You'll also do any preparation, such as tape-recording yourself reading aloud a particular meditation for playback later. (On Day 1 of the program, give yourself a little extra time, as there are six short exercises that will set you up for the entire plan. However, no recording is necessary for Step 1.) On the first day of Step 2, you'll read Chapter 6, including its exercises, and again do any advance work necessary for the week, and so on.

RECORDING THE EXERCISES

On the first day of each step, give yourself some extra time to read the chapter and tape-record the exercises that require you to do so. Some of the activities don't require recording—they can simply be read and then followed. The ones for which you should use a tape are marked (in general, these are longer and more involved).

Recording the instructions will ensure that you can stay present and won't have to turn to the book. You'll also be able to practice with your eyes closed, which will heighten your sensitivity and allow you greater concentration. After you've practiced a particular task with your eyes closed for a period of time and feel that you've mastered it, you can also try it with your eyes open. This will help you translate the gains into your daily life.

Read the guidelines for the exercise into the machine, speaking slowly and clearly. Remember to pause often while reading the instructions to give yourself time to make the internal shifts. Use the same soothing, gentle voice that you would if you were reading to a baby or small child. This is a sound that your inner child can respond to easily. Over time, you won't need the recording anymore because you will have internalized the script.

THE POWER OF WRITING THINGS DOWN

In many of the exercises, you'll be asked to write something down, such as your beliefs, obstacles, or desires. I encourage you to take the time to commit these things to paper, as opposed to simply doing the lesson in your head. There's a certain power that comes from this, and it does impress the teachings upon your subconscious mind. At some points, you'll be coming back to the lists you made earlier, which is all the more reason to write down your responses in a permanent-weight-loss journal that you can refer to again and again.

In addition, take time to make notes about your insights, impressions, and experiences in your permanent-weight-loss journal after each exercise throughout the 40 days. Even if something seems simple or very obvious, it can turn out to be an important key for you later on. Writing down what you've learned and the benefits you've gained is as important as actually doing the work.

GETTING COMFORTABLE

When you sit down to do the exercises, make sure that you're situated in a place where you won't be disturbed for the entire duration of the task. Wear comfortable clothing, make sure that you're in a relaxed position, and turn off your phone. Have your tape player, recording of the exercise for the day, pen, and permanent-weight-loss journal handy so that you can complete the session without interruption. If you wear glasses and don't need them to read the instructions, take them off and play back the tape when you're ready.

USING YOUR IMAGINATION

Some of the instructions include phrases such as *Imagine yourself.* . . . Don't be concerned if you don't "see" anything, because each of us imagines in our own way. You may get clear visuals as if you were watching a movie, or you may instead get a sense of an event occurring. You may have more of a feeling about the event, or there might be a strong auditory component. There's no right or wrong way to use your imagination; be assured that you're imagining all the time. In the exercises that follow, you'll simply be using this skill consciously to create what you truly desire.

Let Go of All Expectations

Try to let go of any ideas about how the exercise should be done. Don't try to force yourself to feel anything; instead, give yourself permission to be exactly where you are and experience it just as it happens. Whatever you're feeling is absolutely fine. Sometimes you may wish to sit down to practice the exercises, and sometimes you may want to stand. Occasionally, you'll feel agitated, distracted, or bored. Just go with it—whether it's bliss and freedom or less pleasant sensations. Say yes to your experience and allow it to be without needing to "fix" it.

Don't try to force yourself to feel love or forgiveness. I assure you that being with your real emotions in the moment creates an opening for natural transformation. As you witness, feel, and experience the turbulence of your passing emotional states, remember that it doesn't mean you have to identify with them. For instance, just because you're feeling anger on a particular day doesn't mean that you're an angry person.

These sensations are transitory, like the weather or the waves of the ocean. Some days the sea is calm, and at other times it's turbulent. But always below the surface is the tranquil, deep Source for those waves—the magnificent, peaceful, life-filled, enormous depths. Let yourself be where you are right now, and commit to doing the exercises regardless of what comes up for you. When you notice that your mind has drifted off, gently come back to your voice on the recording or the written instructions.

STAYING ON TRACK

If, for whatever reason, your emotional state is too strong for the scheduled lesson of the day, feel free to use the awareness exercise in Step 3 instead, if that works better for you. That particular exercise is extremely helpful for relaxing the body and calming the nervous system.

Also, it might be beneficial to change the time of day that you're practicing. If your mind is really racing, it can be challenging to settle into some of the exercises, so be gentle with yourself. If you need to, you can continue when you feel more settled, but don't let stress stop you from following through. Sometimes when life is most difficult, you may actually be the most open to profound learning and internal shifts, and be able to enter into the deeper and more subtle realms of your inner mind, heart, and soul.

If you do miss a day, be sure to get right back on track. Remember, if you're trying to get to New York and your plane is veering toward Houston, just self-correct your course.

As you begin a step, commit to doing each exercise at least once, even those that you aren't drawn to, or which bring up uncomfortable emotions. Then, as you continue to practice for the rest of the week, it's fine to rotate them or repeat the ones that are the most beneficial for you.

Taking Action Daily

While you're doing the inner work of Steps 1 through 6 over the course of 40 days, you'll also need to do the outer work of changing your eating habits. Don't begin the program until after you've read Part I, which will explain how to get going in the right direction.

I don't expect you to change your eating habits in a day or even a week. Start small with the goal of making one significant change each week, such as trying out an unfamiliar food that I recommend or replacing an unhealthy dish with a more nutritious one.

My clients usually find that as they progress with the inner work laid out in the six steps, they don't have to rely on willpower to keep changing their eating behaviors. They actually begin creating new habits from within. So during each week, find three new ideas from Part I that you can implement. It can be as simple as carrying water around with you, eating only half of what's on your plate, or taking the stairs instead of the elevator. By the end of each week, you should have made at least one significant change to your lifestyle. And if you do the same thing every day for the entire program, you'll create a new positive habit!

Connecting with Your Heart

In many of the exercises, you'll be encouraged to connect with your heart. When I refer to this, I'm not speaking of the muscle that beats in your chest, but the core of your being that loves. When I talk about your heart center, I'm not referring to where the physical organ resides, but an area from your throat to your solar plexus, from the front of your chest to your back, and all the space in between, which many spiritual traditions say is where the energy of your heart resides.

If you have trouble connecting to this concept, place your hand on your upper chest, open your mouth, and feel your breath entering and leaving your body through your heart center. Putting your hand on your chest periodically is a wonderful way to bring your attention back to your "deep heart" and all of the resources there.

The heart's energy is enormous: The physical body part has an electromagnetic field 5,000 times greater than that of the brain. And metaphysically, it's the doorway to the world of your highest consciousness and your Creator.

In the exercises that follow, you won't be *thinking* about your heart—you'll be focusing your awareness on this center with an intention to open it. When you set your hand on your chest and place your full conscious awareness there with the intention of connecting to the

Divine within, you'll begin to get a taste of the unconditional love and unity that exists inside you. You really do have to open up to experience this.

How do you open your heart? It's similar to straining in the dark to see something, or craning your neck and opening your hearing to take in the faint sound of music coming from the basement. It's as if you were sniffing deeply to detect a blueberry pie baking next door, while asking yourself *Hmmm, what is that smell?*

The more you practice opening your heart (and being willing to bow your mind to it and put your thinking second), the more the world of the Divine will be revealed to you. This is your true Source of wisdom. You can know full well that you need to exercise and eat fruits and vegetables, but until God makes it possible for your perception of these activities to change, you're hopeless. You can't do it by yourself, but with the help of your inner Source, you can absolutely achieve your goal.

What You'll Do Each Week

Now that you have a better idea of the general practices and theories you'll use, here's an overview of what you'll be doing during each week of the Right Weigh program.

STEP 1: KNOW YOUR VISION, DAYS 1 TO 7

Day 1 only: Read all of Chapter 5, including the instructions for each exercise that you'll be working on at least once (even if you've already read them). There are no exercises that need to be recorded for Step 1. Take whatever time you need to do Exercise 1: Create Your Vision.

- Do Exercise 2: Moving Away from Pain and Toward Pleasure (5 minutes).

- Do Exercise 3: Goal and Strategy Setting (5 minutes).

- Do Exercise 4: Updating Disempowering Beliefs (15 to 30 minutes).

- Do Exercise 5: Create Visual Cues to Reinforce New Beliefs (10 to 15 minutes).

Days 2 to 7: Continue to carry your "Vision Card" with your written outcome on it; mark it and work with it as described in Exercise 1. Continue paying attention to your visual cues, as described in Exercise 5, and try a few new actions from Part I. Make sure to spend ten minutes jotting down in your permanent-weight-loss journal any insights, experiences, or benefits gained while doing the exercises.

Each day, also do at least one of the following exercises:

- Exercise 4: Updating Disempowering Beliefs (15 minutes). Note that you may want to work with different beliefs on different days.

- Exercise 6: Make Mini-Movies of Your Outcome (5 to 10 minutes)

STEP 2: TURN TO YOUR SOURCE FOR HELP, DAYS 8 TO 14

Be sure to set aside extra time on Day 8 to read Chapter 6 and record the exercises for Step 2. Continue working with your Vision Card and visual cues daily, and incorporate at least three new actions from Part I into your life this week.

Each day, write down in your permanent-weight-loss journal any insights, experiences, or benefits you gained from doing the exercises. Also do one of the following lessons:

- Exercise 7: Grounding (10 minutes). Note that you may want to incorporate a short version into the beginning of the other activities that you do in this program.

- Exercise 8: Remembrance (15 to 25 minutes)

- Exercise 9: Bringing in Your Divine Qualities (15 to 20 minutes)

STEP 3: ACCEPT YOURSELF AS YOU ARE, DAYS 15 TO 21

Be sure to set aside extra time on Day 15 to read Chapter 7 and record the exercises for Step 3. Continue working with your Vision Card and visual cues daily, and incorporate at least three new actions from Part I into your life this week.

Each day, write down in your permanent-weight-loss journal any insights, experiences, or benefits you gained from doing the exercises. Each day, do one of the following lessons:

- Exercise 10: Accepting What Is (10 to 20 minutes)
- Exercise 11: Cultivating the Inner Witness (5 minutes)
- Exercise 12: Expanding Your Awareness (10 to 20 minutes)

STEP 4: BREAK FREE FROM OBSTACLES, DAYS 22 TO 28

Be sure to set aside extra time on Day 22 to read Chapter 8 and record the exercises for Step 4. Continue working with your Vision Card and visual cues daily, and incorporate at least three new actions from Part I into your life this week.

Each day, write down in your permanent-weight-loss journal any insights, experiences, or benefits you gained from doing the exercises. Each day, do one of the following lessons:

- Exercise 13: Contacting Your Inner Wisdom (15 to 20 minutes)

- Exercise 14: What Should I Eat? (5 minutes)

- Exercise 15: Silencing the Voices That Hold You Back (15 to 25 min)

- Exercise 16: Healing Through the Voices (10 minutes)

STEP 5: REPROGRAM YOUR SUBCONSCIOUS MIND AND CREATE YOUR FUTURE, DAYS 29 TO 35

Be sure to set aside extra time on Day 29 to reread Chapter 9 and record the exercises for Step 5. Continue working with your Vision Card and visual cues daily, and incorporate at least three new actions from Part I into your life this week.

Each day, write down in your permanent-weight-loss journal any insights, experiences, or benefits you gained from doing the exercises. Each day, do one of the following lessons:

- Exercise 17: Self-Hypnosis to Create Your Future (15 to 20 minutes)

- Exercise 18: Changing Your Perceptions of Pleasure and Pain (5 minutes)

- Exercise 19: Changing Your Internal Pictures (10 minutes)

- Exercise 20: Mental-Movie Reprogramming (5 to 10 minutes)

STEP 6: LETTING GO OF THE PAST, DAYS 36 TO 42

Be sure to set aside extra time on Day 36 to read Chapter 10 and record the exercises for Step 6. Continue working with your Vision Card and visual cues daily, and incorporate at least three new actions from Part I into your life this week.

Each day, write down in your permanent-weight-loss journal any insights, experiences, or benefits you gained from doing the exercises. Each day, do one of the following lessons:

- Exercise 21: Forgiveness (10 minutes)
- Exercise 22: Growing from Mistakes (10 to 15 minutes)
- Exercise 23: Personal Affirmative Prayer (10 to 20 minutes)
- Exercise 24: Prayer to Forgive Yourself (5 minutes)

And now it's time to get started! In the next chapter, you'll begin Step 1—and your journey to freeing yourself from the pain of the past.

CHAPTER FIVE

Step 1: Know Your Vision

What is it that you truly want—that is, what's your vision for your life? In this first step, the most essential element is having a clear image of what you desire. After all, until you can imagine something, how can you achieve it? It's so important to realize that your outer reality is a reflection of your inner beliefs and thoughts about yourself. Do you believe that you deserve to be thin and that you can have a life of happiness and energy? Can you see yourself enjoying meals, yet eating in moderation as a way to gain energy and health? Can you imagine yourself free from food addiction?

The exercises in this chapter will help you answer yes to those questions. As you work through them, you'll be taking an inner journey and moving closer to your goal, freeing yourself from the challenges that have kept you stuck.

Exercise 1: Creating Your Vision

Using your permanent-weight-loss journal, begin writing down your vision for yourself, using the following steps:

1. State your desired outcome in positive, present-tense language (as if it were already happening now). In this way, your subconscious mind can grasp your vision as if it were a command, not just a wish. In other words, rather than "I won't binge at night anymore," it's better to say, "I spend my evenings enjoying activities such as walking or knitting. I am completely satisfied with lemon water and an apple after dinner."

2. Make sure that your outcome is in your control. Don't include sentences such as "My boss never brings doughnuts to work anymore." If your supervisor has supplied morning pastries for the last ten years, he's likely to continue to do so, regardless of your new decisions. A more realistic approach would be: "In every situation, including those at work, I am clear that doughnuts represent the fat on my body and the awful, compulsive, obsessive, out-of-control feeling of addiction. Doughnuts are disgusting to me. I choose to carry healthy, nutritious snacks with me that support the vision I hold for my life: to be healthy, fit, and at my ideal weight."

3. Keep your goal realistic. If your outcome states that you'll lose 30 pounds by the end of next month, you're setting yourself up for failure. Even though you *could* achieve that goal through extreme measures, common sense will tell you that this type of crash dieting can ultimately only take you down the road of failure, and possibly even compromised health. Learn from past mistakes and make your goal absolutely attainable. The experts have always said that slow and steady wins the race. A pound a week is a good, realistic goal—it may not sound like much, but it's the way to keep excess weight off over the long term.

4. Make your outcome measurable and specific, with a time limit. Human beings thrive on working toward some kind of goal. If yours isn't specific or measurable—for instance, if it's simply "I want to lose weight"—that doesn't program any incentive to act now into your very literal subconscious. If your goal is worded as some distant, vague wish, then that's how your mind will respond to it, so write a sense of urgency into your stated vision. If you want to lose 50 pounds and you know that the only way to achieve permanent results is by taking off one pound per week, then plan to meet your goal one year from today.

5. Write down the benefits of attaining your goal. Why are you doing this? Take a moment and fantasize about how much better your life will be when you're actually free from food addiction and its horrible consequences. You'll look and feel better, have more energy, and be free from this emotional prison. You'll be more comfortable, and your health will most likely improve . . . perhaps more than you could have dreamed. Some people who lose weight are surprised by all the unexpected benefits: Allergies and aches and pains mysteriously disappear, blood pressure is reduced, there's less need for medication, and even chronic headaches often vanish. In addition, you'll no longer have to worry about imminent diabetes or heart disease. It's important for you to write down, and look forward to, all of the personal benefits you can expect.

Now it's time for you to refine your vision, keeping in mind the points that you just read. Don't read any further until you've taken this crucial step, which will help you reprogram your beliefs and habits. Remember that your subconscious mind is like a computer on autopilot. Unless you enter in the data that you're determined to achieve, your brain will keep producing the same results, which have led to your present overweight condition and state of health. You want your mind to get the message of your new commitment for your life loud and clear.

Here's an example of a specific vision that follows the five steps for creating your outcome as outlined above:

> I, Rena Greenberg, am 115 pounds by April 2007. I enjoy in-line skating once or twice a week and taking regular walks. I love to eat salad with protein and flaxseed oil, along with some complex carbohydrates. I feel fantastic and have lots of energy. I am free of any sugar addiction, no matter what situation I am in. I love the way my new body looks and feels. I am filled with gratitude for the strength and courage to achieve my vision. And I relax easily with prayer and meditation.

Create and refine your vision for your life now. After you've written it down in your journal, take a moment to move through time to your target date and imagine this new reality. Take it in with all of your senses as you picture yourself and your life in this completely new way. This goal isn't a simple wish, but a heartfelt decision that you're now changing your life for the better. You're choosing the higher road for the rest of the time that you have here on this planet.

Begin watching a Technicolor internal video of this new reality that you're stepping into, and make it very real. Envision yourself living at your target weight and feeling fabulous, happy, and peaceful; loving the way you eat now; choosing healthy dishes; leaving food on your plate naturally; only eating when you're physically hungry; and really enjoying your new, increased activity level.

Once you've scripted your positive mental movie, keep playing it. In fact, try to get emotional about it so that it has more of an impact. Really experience the joy and pleasure as you see this movie in your mind! Remember, if you hadn't played so many scenes about how fabulous chocolate cake tastes and the joy of eating it (versus the painful deprivation of eating rice, steamed vegetables, or other "diet" food), you wouldn't have been able to successfully create an overweight condition either.

Remember: *Write the goal, then speak and hear it.* Use all your senses and strong emotions to truly make a strong impression on your brain. Every time you do, it's as if you're pushing a button on a computer and entering this new program.

After you've done the writing and envisioning, copy your desired outcome from your journal onto an index card. Keep it in your purse or pocket where you can get to it easily throughout the day. Every time you do something that supports your desired outcome, put a mark on the front of the card; whenever you do something that sabotages yourself, put a mark on the back of the card.

The purpose of this exercise is to help you to acknowledge all your positive actions and to become aware of what's self-defeating. Much of your limiting behavior is automatic, so this will help you see more clearly any problem areas that you can work on in the later chapters. Tell yourself that every time you have 20 (or any number you determine) positive marks on the front side of the card, you'll reward yourself with something you really enjoy (not food)—such as a massage, theater tickets, a mini-vacation, a new outfit, taking an interesting class, and so on.

Creating your vision and checking in every day to see if your behavior is supporting or sabotaging it is so important that I urge you to do this throughout the 40 days of the program (creating new index cards, as necessary). Each day when you read your vision to yourself, imagine that it's actually true for you now, in the present moment. Use all your senses to make the imagery vivid and real.

Exercise 2: Moving Away from Pain and Toward Pleasure

Once you're really clear about the vision for your life, you need to begin to associate pleasure with those behaviors that will bring you to your goal, and pain with the actions that don't.

Humans naturally move away from pain and toward pleasure. Let that discomfort motivate you to make a decision to change old, unproductive behaviors into ones that will lead to the results you want. Then you can focus on the excitement of losing weight and keeping it off.

The point of becoming aware of this suffering isn't to feel guilty about the situation you're in now or to reinforce the fact that you're helpless and out of control around food. That only serves to make you feel bad and continue to recycle the old, negative eating habits. Instead, the point is to make the connection in your mind right now between the anguish that you're in and your automatic, unproductive eating behaviors that are causing that heartache. This can be a strong motivator to help you change.

To achieve the success you desire, you need to truly acknowledge the pain that your current situation causes you—and anticipate the pleasure that you're moving toward.

USING THE PLEASURE-PAIN PRINCIPLE FOR YOUR BENEFIT

Whatever your subconscious association of pleasure and pain, you can learn to change them. One of the main obstacles to achieving and maintaining your ideal weight is your pleasurable associations with the "wrong" foods. Somewhere in your mind, you have many links between food and rewards, satisfaction, and being sociable. For instance, if you have these good feelings for items that are oily, greasy, and salty, you can use your willpower to stay away from them for a period of time, but sooner or later—usually under stress—you'll go toward that source of pleasure again.

Similarly, if you associate pain with working out, yet you've chosen joining a fitness center as your way of doing exercise, then even though you can use willpower and drag yourself to the gym for a while, at some point you'll declare that it's just too difficult, and you'll move away from this source of unhappiness.

To maximize your potential for change, you'll need to really feel the pain associated with your current weight condition and eating habits so that you feel compelled to move away from it. Where are you going to be in five years if you continue with your lifestyle the way it is? How about ten years? Take a moment and notice how your body feels: Are you constantly tired, lethargic, or sick? Do you need stimulants such as sugar, white flour, caffeine, prescription drugs, or alcohol to get you through the day? Is this the way you want to keep living, thereby destroying your health? Let these sensations motivate you to say, "I've had enough." Those magic words will change your life, especially when there are strong emotions behind them.

If you feel that your life is going pretty well except for this issue of food addiction and/or being overweight, and you really don't relate to the concept of being in anguish, think about all the time you spend on food obsessions, dieting intermittently, health concerns, and generally worrying or thinking about your weight and/or health. Even if you aren't in actual physical or emotional pain, wouldn't it be nice to free up this huge chunk of your life and begin fulfilling your life's purpose? Can you imagine what it would be like to have a deeper connection with your own heart and soul and live from this place? What would it be like if you were no longer addicted to particular foods and were in control of your life and eating habits?

Once you've identified the pain, start focusing on pleasure. You're much more likely to reach your goal when you start to move toward the satisfaction of living life healthy, fit, and in control of your life and your eating habits. You need to imagine yourself becoming slender and maintaining that shape. It's imperative that you feel the bliss of your ideal weight *before* you achieve it, as if you were already there. When you clearly imagine what you want, you're on your way to creating that in your outer reality.

The subconscious mind doesn't differentiate between what's real and imagined; imagination creates reality. It's not necessarily your wishes that come true, but your predominant thoughts and your expectations. Because you're simply running on autopilot 95 percent of the time, if you do something and it feels good, you'll end up repeating it. If it feels bad, however, you'll naturally avoid it. Also, when you imagine something while experiencing a strong emotion, such as fear or excitement, your subconscious mind actually begins to send out impulses to make you feel like engaging in the very behavior you're imagining.

Take some time to answer the following questions, and write down your answers in your permanent-weight-loss journal:

- What pain motivates you?

- What will it cost you personally if you don't take charge of your life and your eating habits now?

- What pleasure are you moving toward?

WAYS TO SWITCH PLEASURE AND PAIN ASSOCIATIONS

Whether you're addicted to eating a bag of chips every day after work or running two miles, either way your brain is using a program that was installed at some point, and you can choose to overwrite it with a new one. When you do that, your habits will change. If you start scripting and directing a movie of just how fatigued you'll feel after work tomorrow and how exhausting it will be to drag yourself to the gym, this powerful emotional image you've created for yourself will manifest.

On the other hand, if you imagine that you'll put on your headphones and take a run outside, smelling the fresh, clean air and feeling your limbs pumping to the beat of the music, that's what you'll re-create instead.

Similarly, if you constantly tell yourself, "I'm so fat, and I have no willpower—nothing works for me!" you're making it impossible for those conditions to change. For instance, at first it may seem unnatural for you to reach for water instead of diet soda when you're thirsty. However, when you make the choice to read about the chemicals in sugar-free beverages and realize the possible harm inherent in these products, it becomes easier to make a decision to break that habit. When you learn that there are many studies to show that chemicals such as aspartame may actually stimulate hunger or cravings for sugar, you can intellectually decide to make a new choice. But what about your repeated happy associations with drinking diet soda?

Step back and realize that your attachment to certain foods and beverages is simply a result of the current programming in your brain. If, on the other hand, you made the conscious decision to drink water throughout the day and walk two miles after lunch, then all you'd need to do is install a different program and these activities would begin to feel natural. At first, of course, the new behavior will probably seem awkward; but if you run mental movies of drinking pure water and feeling refreshed, and of really enjoying that walk and all of its benefits, you'll soon reprogram your subconscious to experience these activities as pleasurable.

So picture yourself walking as you listen to your favorite music or reciting positive affirmations as you enjoy the fresh air and scenery. Imagine that you now love it so much that you walk, rain or shine, simply adjusting your clothing depending on the weather. Consciously choose the course of action that you want, because the dominant program in your brain is determining your behavior.

As soon as you realize that you're focusing on a negative image of yourself as overweight and out of control, change that image to what you truly do want to create: a new life; enjoying a healthy, fit body; happy and in control. Remember that it's your dominant, consistent thoughts that create your reality—particularly when these thoughts are fueled by strong emotion.

Typically, when you aren't using your mind's capacity to serve yourself, but instead are using it to hurt yourself, you might spend all day imagining how good something will taste (anticipating pleasure), then eat it . . . and feel the pain or guilt of what it's doing to your body or how it makes you feel. What you can learn to do instead is reverse this process—before you eat this particular food, you'll feel the discomfort it's going to bring you, which will diminish any cravings for it.

By doing this, you can avoid much of the self-sabotage and guilt that may have become so routine in your life. When the deeply ingrained pleasure-pain principle that's hardwired into your brain is harnessed and utilized for your own benefit, you can transform it from causing a predictable pattern of failure into a sure means for success.

Exercise 3: Goal and Strategy Setting

Your vision gives you your long-term goal and reminds you of why it's so important to have the better life you dream of. Setting short-term goals and coming up with a strategy for reaching them helps ensure that you get there. Studies actually show that people who write down their desires are much more likely to achieve them than people who merely think about them. Writing things down is a great way to impress them upon the subconscious mind.

But what good is a goal without a strategy for reaching it? What are the actual steps you're committing to? The bottom line is that the only way to lose weight is to take in less food than you're burning off. It's that simple. It doesn't matter if you aren't eating any more than you did ten years ago or that your neighbor puts away three times as much as you do. In order to succeed, you need to be honest with yourself and start envisioning a realistic strategy that will get you where you want to go. Use the tips from Part I to help you create a strategy and action plan that will work for you.

In this exercise, you'll begin to write down your specific goals and the steps that you intend to take to reach them. After you've done the Right Weigh program, update this chart on a monthly basis.

5.1 GOAL-SETTING CHART						
	Jan.	Feb.	Mar.	Apr.	May	June
My current weight is:						
My goal for this month:						
Strategy:						

Exercise 4: Updating Disempowering Beliefs

Now that you're very clear about your outcome and goals, it's time to look at any beliefs that are working against you. Your expectations are based on what you hold to be true, and because you're set on automatic pilot, the resulting behavior is often self-destructive. The good news is that this can be altered, and that's what this exercise will help you do.

Begin by taking out your journal or a sheet of paper. At the top, label it: Beliefs about My Ability to Lose Weight Permanently. Think about what you consider true about your ability to achieve your ideal weight. Some common unproductive core assumptions are:

- I'll always be fat.
- I have no willpower.
- I love chocolate.

GOAL-SETTING CHART cont'd.						
	July	Aug.	Sept.	Oct.	Nov.	Dec.
My current weight is:						
My goal for this month:						
Strategy:						

- I don't have time to exercise.
- I'll never find the time to cook.
- My family situation won't allow me to change my eating habits over the long term.
- I have no control.
- I have to take care of everybody else first.
- This is going to be so hard.
- I just want everything to be easy.
- I hate not eating whatever I want.
- If I don't eat certain foods, I'll feel deprived.
- If I didn't overeat, my emotions would be out of control.
- It's in my genes to be overweight.
- My parents caused this.
- Healthy food tastes awful.

- I just want to eat what I enjoy.
- I don't really take in that much.
- Thin people can have anything they want and never gain weight.
- I can't exercise.
- My hormones are causing this.
- Even if I don't like it, being heavy gives me a sense of security.

Look through the list above and find any statements that resonate for you. Then spend a few moments reflecting on other core ideas you hold regarding your weight and self-image. Without judgment, write them down in your journal.

Now you're going to go down your list and examine it as if you were a scientist. Take each item and write it down at the top of a blank sheet of paper, and then answer the following questions about it:

1. What is the origin of this belief? (If you aren't sure, guess.)

2. What pictures or voices am I aware of when I tune in to this statement?

3. Did either of my parents (or caregivers or role models) carry this same idea about me or about themselves?

4. Is this an absolute truth? Is it unchangeable or irreversible?

5. Does this serve me? Is it useful in any way?

6. What would be a more empowering belief?

This process may bring up uncomfortable feelings, and the old assumption may not want to die without a fight. Don't let that concern you. Just keep your eyes on your vision, knowing that this is how you'll achieve it. Don't focus your attention on what you don't want anymore.

You may notice that you're attached to the idea that your beliefs are true or right. After examining them, it's important to replace each one with a more empowering statement, even if the new idea isn't truthful yet. Decide which values, decisions, and strategies will give you the life you want.

For example, let's say you wrote: "I *love* to eat." Your new constructive belief may be: "I love to eat the foods that nourish me and support me." If you believe: "Healthy food tastes awful," then your new, empowering affirmation might be: "I choose to eat healthy foods that are absolutely delicious and bursting with flavor. I am completely turned off by repulsive, greasy stuff that is poisonous to my system."

The more senses and strong emotions you use as you create these new statements, the more likely your subconscious mind is to buy in to them. For instance, you might want to recall the most revolting image of being overweight or overeating that you can, or a time when you felt very empowered by being in control, and use this to create a strong conviction that you can install on a deeper level. As you examine your old ideas, remember that the bottom line is whether the concepts you hold serve you, not whether they're true.

You'll be well rewarded for the time that you put into this exercise because you'll achieve a heightened level of consciousness. So go ahead and shine the light of your awareness on each negative belief and expose it for the lie it is.

I hope that this is an exercise you'll work with not just during the 40-day program, but afterward, because repetition is the key to success. From now on, whenever the old belief pops up in any shape or form, immediately wipe it out by repeating the new one.

Whether your subconscious mind accepts this fresh idea and manifests new results in your life also depends on your commitment to act as if it's true even as you continue to reprogram your mind. Remember that the only reason the old one seems true is because you've focused on it so much that your whole outer reality confirms it. You can see that it's become a vicious circle and a self-fulfilling prophecy, and your task is to stop that hurtful process!

As you stay with this, you may discover that other old, unproductive beliefs begin to surface. Take the time to identify them and go through the above exercise with each one, writing it down and answering the series of questions about it.

Exercise 5: Create Visual Cues to Reinforce New Beliefs

This exercise is designed to help you focus on your new, positive beliefs as much as you can by using visual reminders that you can look at throughout the course of the day. Making and placing these signs around your environment will have a tremendous impact on your subconscious mind. Notice how effective visual advertising is: The messages you see are embedded in your consciousness. If you want fast and long-lasting results, take the time to make these signs, even if the whole idea seems silly. You'll be astounded as these new beliefs begin to take hold in your brain and your behaviors start to change effortlessly. Here's what to do:

1. **Write each of your new, empowering beliefs on sticky notes and place them everywhere**—such as in your bathroom, car, or bedroom; and on the refrigerator. You might include any of your new empowering beliefs, such as: "It feels great to move my body" or "I reach for water throughout the day."

2. **Put up photos of yourself at your ideal weight.** If you don't have any, find a picture of someone with your body type. Make sure it's realistic, put your face on the photo, and then put the image where you can see it on a regular basis.

3. **Focus on your new belief throughout your day.** Bring your positive ideas to mind first thing in the morning and at night when you're falling asleep, when your subconscious is most open to suggestion.

4. **Repeat the productive beliefs to yourself when you're driving, brushing your teeth, showering, or taking out the trash.** Don't just say the words to yourself silently—say them aloud, if you can.

5. **Each time you repeat the productive belief, bring in strong emotions and your other senses to strengthen the message to your subconscious.** Bring in your other senses and your emotions to help you. If one of your reminders is "I love steamed vegetables with brown rice," imagine the smell and taste of it as you say it, and then visualize that food on your plate. If your cue is "I feel good when I've eaten a meal and my stomach is not quite full," imagine that pleasant, not-stuffed sensation.

Exercise 6: Make Mini-Movies of Your Outcome

To create the behaviors you truly desire, take a few moments to go through this list of possible, positive outcomes for you. Next, write down in your journal some of the specific outcomes you want, for example:

My desired outcome is to . . .

- Fit into my clothes comfortably.
- Look and feel my best.
- Be free from food addiction.
- Be in control of my life and my eating habits.
- Like my reflection in the mirror.
- Be comfortable in my body.
- Eat only when I'm physically hungry.
- Be naturally attracted to the foods that bring me health and energy.
- Love myself fully.
- Truly appreciate and honor the gift of my life.
- Take care of my physical body.
- Nurture myself in healthy ways.
- Have inner peace even in stressful situations.

Now, look at each positive outcome that you wrote down, and imagine what it would be like if this were actually true for you now. It may be easier for you to create and reinforce your vision for yourself if you actually see it playing like a mini-movie in your mind, as I mentioned in Exercise 1. If you're not quite sure what outcome you want, this exercise can help you solidify it. So create a Technicolor mini-movie of yourself engaging in the positive behaviors that will lead to your desired outcomes.

For example, if you're stopped at a traffic light and are feeling hungry—and you spy a fast-food drive-through—play the "repulsive-burger/delicious-salad-at-home" scenario. When you're walking through a shopping mall looking at clothes on display, play a different inspiring part from the DVD of your new reality. Here are some more scenes that might be a part of your story:

- You eat only when you are truly, physically hungry.

- You hear your own inner dialogue supporting and congratulating you in a soothing, upbeat, nurturing voice as you make healthy choices. You see a rich, sugary, buttery food and feel repulsed. You're disgusted by such empty calories that are harmful to your system and push them away from you. Then a plate of nutritious, healthy food that smells heavenly is in front of you. You take a bite and savor its taste and texture.

- Feeling energized by the good food you ate, you're exercising and enjoying the movement of your body. You're dancing, in-line skating, running, biking, playing tennis, or jumping on a trampoline. You feel so good about yourself!

- You're at a birthday party for your nephew, repulsed by the cake with its greasy, chemical-laden, fatty frosting, and you're enjoying talking with people instead of forcing yourself to eat a piece just for show.

Congratulations! You've made it through the first step of the Right Weigh program. Remember to keep doing the exercises that work for you as you move on to the next step in Chapter 6.

CHAPTER SIX

Step 2: Turn to Your Source for Help

Do you eat as a way to avoid painful feelings, give love to yourself, and fill a deep void? Unfortunately, reaching for a snack as a way to fulfill yourself is one of the greatest obstacles to achieving permanent weight loss.

Food that tastes good is something that has literally filled you. When you're indulging in a delicious treat, you feel happy. However, because this joy is temporary and illusory, you experience disappointment over and over again—your mind doesn't see any alternative and seeks to be satisfied with the fleeting pleasures of taste sensations. In the meantime, your internal pit of frustration is growing.

When you're inevitably disappointed by the people around you, or your life situation, you may try harder to change your outer circumstances—or just reach for food to satisfy your emptiness and soothe your pain. What is it that you really, truly need, in the deepest place in your heart and soul? (Hint: It isn't more food!)

Stop Using Food to Fill a Void

The vacuum inside that you seek to stuff with food can only be filled with Divine love: the unconditional, deep, profound presence that's at the core of all existence. It's the field of oneness that many experience in nature or a moment of awe or bliss.

Most people are disconnected from this higher reality the majority of the time. This feeling of separation, which they may not even be aware of, causes them to act self-destructively. Eating to stop this yearning and obsessing over food keeps them from feeling and knowing the real energy that's at the core of their being.

In this chapter, you'll rediscover the ocean of Divine love, safety, and wisdom that's available to you with every breath you take. As you tap in to this inexhaustible inner resource, you'll finally be able to stop using food as a way to suppress any wounds dwelling inside you and find comfort. You'll begin to eat the way you were meant to—as a means of staying alive and nourishing your body.

An Eternal, Inexhaustible Resource

This Source of unlimited creativity, wisdom, love, knowledge, and power that you'll be contacting is what many people refer to as God. Most of us were never taught to relate to this vast, unlimited Source in a personal way. Not only is it possible to do so, but when you do, you'll receive insight and guidance that is far more valuable than what you could have obtained with your intellect alone. You'll be uplifted and your life will be re-created, and you'll probably long to enhance your communication with your personal Source.

You may have felt so disconnected from the Source of deep love within your heart that you doubt whether such a love even exists. I assure you that a bounty of Divine love and happiness is available to you in any given moment. Although it may be completely clouded over because you're distracted by other thoughts and emotions, it nonetheless exists as an eternal resource for true peace, joy, strength, and protection. When you're in an airplane flying through thick clouds, you may have no evidence of the sun, yet you know that it's always there. In the same way, no matter what's happening in your outer life, if you dig deep enough you'll find an innate awareness that you aren't alone. You're an inseparable part of an infinite field of unity, which is patiently waiting for you to return.

Look Inward, Not Outward

If you're like most overweight people, you've tried every diet that's come down the pike, read every new health book that's been released, and followed more exercise regimens than you care to remember. Consequently, you may be conditioned to think that there's help out-side of you: some "expert" out there who can outline a specific meal plan or get you to exercise regularly and vigorously. While it's possible that there is someone who has the answers you seek, is there any person who can motivate you from the *inside* to follow through? Is there any human being who can completely change your thoughts and beliefs so that you'll lose weight naturally and easily? Is there someone who can transform you so that you think and behave like a thin person for the rest of your life? It's highly unlikely that you'll ever find such a person.

So where can you find the help you need? You can discover it only within yourself, with your Creator who resides inside your heart. Deep within your core is a holy jewel: your essence, which was placed there by God. Once you begin to get in touch with the truth of who you are, you can receive inner guidance on how to proceed in order to achieve the outcome you desire. As a beautiful, Divine gem, you deserve the highest level of respect. You need to honor the vessel—the body—that houses your Divine soul.

The answers truly are inside of you and nowhere else. Sure, you can read a lot about the benefits of healthy foods, the value of the glycemic index, the perils of carbohydrates, the dangers of fat or animal protein, the pros and cons of calorie counting, and the benefits of various types of exercise—yet it's really up to you to determine which foods and behaviors support you and which don't. Only you can arrange your life to incorporate the activities that work for you, that you enjoy, and that you can comfortably fit into your busy schedule.

Now before any despair starts to creep in, realize that you don't have to figure out everything on your own or stay motivated all by yourself, using only your conscious mind, which is analytical and intel-ligent but limited. If you could achieve your goal of living healthy and fit at your ideal weight by yourself, you would have done it by now, right? You need help, and you can get it from the huge, eternal, inexhaustible Source of wisdom, strength, and power within yourself.

You may ask, "If this Source exists within me, where has it been for the last 30 years?" The answer is that it's been there protecting and loving you, although you may not have been aware of it. God is always inside of you, but you've been given free will. You must choose to stop and ask for the help you desire and need. When you do so humbly and patiently, your prayers will be answered.

Sometimes it takes practice to hear and notice the subtle voice of your Creator. This is what you'll be doing in the exercises in this chapter.

Turning to Your Source Regularly

It's natural to feel skeptical about the power of your inner Source on some level. Perhaps you already practice meditation and feel that you do have an active communication with your Creator but it hasn't made your problem disappear. I assure you that the exercises you're going to do will help you be more aware of this Power; and the more often you do them, the easier they'll be.

Perhaps you experienced an awareness of your Source on a very special day, such as the birth of your baby, your wedding, or even the death of a loved one. Well, have you ever had an experience of *complete* love and peace? Have you ever felt as if time simply stopped and you were connected to everyone and everything; and you could literally hear, feel, see, taste, and smell the deep miracle of the tapestry of life? If you have, know that this experience isn't meant to be a rare event. You aren't supposed to only check in with your Source occasionally when you say a prayer or try meditation. You're intended to live and commune with the Most High regularly.

Once you have a closer relationship with the One who is making you breathe and keeping you alive, you'll find it easier to tune in to the vast levels of personal guidance available. Your inner wisdom will assist you on your journey to health, your ideal weight, and the greater purpose for your life.

You may be unsure whether it's really all that important to connect with your inner Source, and wonder whether this part of the program makes sense for you. I assure you that it's the foundation upon which all of the other steps rest. In my experience, you can only end your overweight condition forever by surrendering the entire problem to your Creator on a regular basis and watching as your new life, thoughts, and behaviors begin to unfold.

Whether or not you believe in God, if you were on a sinking ship, who would you call out to? Call out to that One now, and let your life be made new and whole.

Exercise 7: Grounding

Even though God is everywhere, we connect to this power through the body and most specifically through the heart. You might be astounded to realize how much time you spend in your head completely cut off from the rest of yourself (unless you're experiencing some physical pain). Grounding allows you to fully connect with your physical self. It's through your body that you can reach the depths of Spirit within you and therefore create the greatest internal shifts. This exercise also helps you expand your awareness beyond the limitations of thinking alone by putting you in touch with your greater nature. And it helps you constantly be reminded of the steadfast support the earth is here to give you, even if you've never stopped to notice that before.

Record This Exercise

Close your eyes and become aware of your breath coming in and out of your nose and mouth. Feel your breath travel into your lungs. Feel it moving through your lungs and entering your bloodstream, bringing oxygen and nutrients to every cell of your body.

Direct your attention to the area in your body about three inches below your navel and halfway between the front of your belly and the small of your back. Focus your awareness here, the area that many Eastern traditions consider to be your power center. Take your time and sense this place deep inside your lower abdomen. Tune in to this source of power.

As you become aware of it, imagine that in the center of your belly there's a ball of fire, something within you that you can draw strength from. Imagine that there's a cord attached to this blaze that travels down through your body, through the floor, into the ground, through the layers of the earth, and down into the molten core of the world.

As you feel the connection that is being made between the center of the earth and your own power center, start to focus your awareness on your legs. Imagine that they have roots spreading deep into the earth, supporting you and bringing you energy and vitality. Feel the strength and power of the soil as you make contact in this way. Allow yourself to receive the support that the earth has to give you.

Give yourself permission to relax and make contact with this center of power inside yourself. Stand up and feel your legs. Take your time as you allow your consciousness to descend to the lower part of your body. Let your breath drop down into your abdomen and feel its rise and fall there. As you do so, sense this internal source of strength.

Feel your legs reaching down deep into the earth again. Notice how strong you are . . . how solid you are. Stand tall and connect with your power.

When you're ready, gently open your eyes and come back into the room.

This exercise is so useful and powerful that you may want to do it (or a shorter version) before you try other activities—particularly if you're having trouble getting out of your head.

Unexpected Blessings and Joy

When you do at last surrender to the great Divine Force within you and allow yourself to receive its blessings, you'll experience a sweetness and relief that will fill you from the very depths of your being. It will be as if every cell of your body is opening to allow a soothing, fragrant nectar to infuse it. You'll almost be able to hear the fibers of your being relaxing with relief: "Aaaah!"

As you delight in this experience, you may think, *If it was so simple, why did I wait so long?* In the classic film *The Wizard of Oz*, when Dorothy asked the good witch Glinda why she didn't tell her before she began her journey that all she had to do to go home was click her heels three times and keep repeating "There's no place like home," the witch gave her the answer: "Because you wouldn't have believed me."

The same is probably true for you. Like so many people, you needed to go through your struggles to arrive at a place where you could be receptive to surrendering to the only Source that can truly give you what you want. The incident that motivated you to take this journey to weight loss may have been something that was the last straw or such a blow that you said, "I'm really ready to change."

Sometimes you need to suffer in order to be jolted out of the stupor you may have been living in . . . and into the life that you're meant to live. At the time, these "hits" can seem like the greatest tragedy, such as illness, the death of a loved one, financial loss, or divorce. But many people who follow this journey actually begin feeling grateful for their past chronic difficulties with their weight and health, because these challenges led them to a point where the suffering was so great that they were finally willing to surrender to something even greater. Because they spent so long searching in vain for answers to their dilemma in the outer world, they were willing to look in the most unlikely place: the deep well of love and beauty inside. What a blessing!

Don't Escape—Connect!

You may find yourself eating as a way to escape from the outer material world, which is so compelling and real that it can be overwhelming. You get caught up in it, and understandably so. It's helpful to take time every day to remember that there are deeper realities beyond the physical world that you take in with your five senses. When you begin to experience these deeper realities, you no longer need to use food to help you escape from this limited existence. Rather than escape, you can connect to your Creator who put you here. When you turn to this Source for comfort, compassion, guidance, and strength in living your life in the highest way possible, you'll truly want to honor your body.

You aren't alone, yet much unconscious eating stems from a deep fear that you are. The Source of love is closer than anything else, yet how many people spend their lives searching for it? You *are* that love! Even if you feel cut off from it, it's within you and you can connect to it. When you feel this link, your desire to care for your body will effortlessly well up from deep inside.

Remember a time when you were in love and how magical it was? All of a sudden, you felt that you didn't need to sleep or eat because you were sustained by this emotion. That power is who you are. You don't need to feel it only once every 20 years and then go back to sleep—you can live from this place.

You may wonder why you often feel completely disconnected from any sense of love. How can it be true that you have access to such a vast body of wisdom and strength if you can feel so alone, troubled, and out of control around food?

When you consistently choose processed foods that are devoid of any nutritional content, the effect on your whole system is to numb you so that it becomes much more difficult to link to your essence. Connecting with the highest unconditional love of your Creator is something that you can only know by doing it. Could you adequately describe the flavor of a crisp, tart Granny Smith apple to someone who's never tasted anything like it? It would be challenging. By the same token, the only way to know what it's like to reach a vast presence far greater than yourself and commune with it regularly is to have a direct experience.

Exercise 8: Remembrance

The ancient Sufi practice of Remembrance may be simple, but it has tremendous power—and the more you perform it, the greater and more profound its effect will be. When you attempt this, all you have to do is repeat the name of your Higher Power, which connects you to that Source within. What you "remember" in this exercise is your deeper nature . . . which it's easy to forget about or lose sight of during the course of daily living.

You'll be repeating the name of God with your tongue but also in your heart. In fact, the most important aspect of the exercise is speaking from your soul with sincerity. When you repeat the name, you aren't uttering a mantra; you're invoking the light of the Most High. So when you're saying it, it's best to also see the name written in light within you, surrounded with the highest, brightest light that you can imagine.

One of the most important aspects of Remembrance is receiving. As best you can during the following exercise, open yourself to receiving the love and blessings that will come to you.

Whatever name for God you use during your practice, it will help you access your own connection to all of life. Your heart is the doorway to this place of oneness, which lies beneath all the differences of personalities, religions, politics, race, and nationality.

Depending on your cultural background, you may want to use a name like Yahweh, Allah, Allahut, Brahman, Adonai, or Elohim. These words come from ancient, sacred languages such as Latin, Sanskrit, Aramaic, Arabic, and Hebrew. The benefit is that each of these contains either the short "a" or long "aaah" sound, which energetically help you open the heart center of your body. It's thought that sacred languages have a power beyond just the meaning of their words— that they actually have a healing, vibrational effect on our bodies. This is why many believe that for meditation, it's important to use a Sanskrit mantra as opposed to an English word.

If, after trying them out, none of these words are comfortable for you, you can try "God," "Spirit," "Divine Oneness," "Divine Love," "Universal Love," "Beloved Lord," "Universal Wisdom," or "One Love." Feel the various effects on your body, and settle for the word or phrase that you feel the most positive energy from physically. If there's no such effect, it's fine to simply say "Aaaah."

Record This Exercise

Close your eyes. Take a deep breath and hold it. . . . now let it out slowly, slowly . . . allowing any tension to leave your body with the breath. And take one more nice, big, deep breath and hold it . . . and exhale, allowing any remaining tension to leave your body with the breath. Take a moment to stretch your arms and hands and legs. Shake them out a little and let your whole body rest and relax.

Place your hand on your upper chest and imagine that as you inhale and exhale, you have two nostrils under your hand in the center of your heart. Bow your head slightly. . . . Allow your focus to shift to your heart as you continue to breathe.

Choose the name of God that you're most comfortable with and begin to repeat it both with your tongue and in your heart center. As you say it very slowly, allow the name to float on your every breath. Imagine it written in light and surrounded by a halo of dazzling brilliance. See it deep in your heart. With every breath you take, breathe in through the imaginary nostrils in your heart, and pull the name deeper into your center. . . . As you utter God's name, sense your profound connection to your Creator. . . . Say the name. . . . Sense the link to your Source within yourself.

If there's no name for God that you're comfortable with at this time, simply keep your hand on your heart and just breathe in and out of your chest. With each exhalation, slowly say "Aaaaaah . . . aaaah."

Remember to slow down your breathing. Notice the internal shift as you focus on your heart. Feel your mind quieting down. If your mind is still racing, that's okay. Just say the name of God . . . watch it go into your heart and then expand and fill your whole being.

As you speak, invoking your Source, keep seeing the name deep within your heart, illuminated. Feel the vibration of the word deep in your chest and hear your own voice, barely audible, as you repeat it to yourself.

Sink down onto your chair or bed, and keep breathing this word deep into your heart. Each time, bring it further inside. Allow each repetition to go deeper than the one before. If you haven't already, place your hand on your chest to help maintain your focus.

Still see the name that you're using written in light across your chest. Drink in this luminescence with each breath. This glow changes and transforms you. In a sense, the light and the name wash your heart clean. If any pictures and voices come into your awareness, just let the name and the light act like a great eraser, wiping them away.

As you repeat God's name, know that you're being blessed. You may feel light . . . expansive . . . relaxed. Notice this sensation and drink it in. . . . Be open to receiving these gifts with sincerity and gratitude. In silence now, continue speaking the name until it's time for you to return to the room. . . .

Take your time with the exercise and be patient. Practice repeating and breathing the name deeper into your heart center until you
experience an internal shift, perhaps like a sinking, heavy feeling, or
maybe a lightness or an opening of your awareness as you connect
to your Source. If you don't feel any of these sensations, it's okay. You
may just need more practice. Be very gentle with yourself.

Keep in mind that it's important to use a name for your Creator
that you're comfortable with. If you wish to intensify your experience,
I encourage you to experiment with another name for God, especially
one with the "Aaah" sound in it. You may notice a substantial difference in the effect when you use a word that naturally opens your
heart with that vibration.

The Remembrance is the basis for some of the other work you'll
be doing to move into a place of freedom, true happiness, and a
healthy life at your ideal weight. The important point to realize is that
this is an exercise in receiving. You're probably wonderful at giving,
but you must remember that it is not selfish to be on the other end.

When you practice Remembrance on a regular basis, you'll receive
love and light directly from your Creator. You'll no longer need to
search for that nurturing from the outer world and from what you eat.
As your personal connection with God becomes stronger, you'll find it
easier to get guidance on the weight and food issues that have been
the most challenging for you. The addictions you clung to before will
easily be released as you learn to fill yourself up with Divine love.

Cleaning Your Heart

When you came into this world, you were steeped in love, innocence, and purity. As you got older, your natural state got covered
over by painful experiences that were locked away inside of you. Any
subsequent suffering, and your interpretations of these events, were
stacked on top of the earlier unresolved traumas.

These memories keep you from experiencing the bliss that's your
birthright. You might even start to think that no such ecstatic love
or God even exists. However, as you clean your heart, you'll start to
reconnect with the Divine qualities of mercy, peace, compassion,

safety, and love within your very own being. The conscious and unconscious pain can be washed away—it's only the residue of the collective anguish in your life that clouds you from truly experiencing an infinite and rich Source that connects you to all of creation. Babies hold this innocence, love, and sense of connectedness very strongly, which is why many people are so attracted to them.

I promise that no matter how clouded over they are, the qualities of oneness, safety, and caring are still within you. As you work with the exercises and cleanse your heart, not only will you free yourself from your obsession with food, but you'll also open up to a whole new world. You'll finally be able to relax in your own skin and get direction from the deep wisdom that lives within you. You'll come to realize that when you get in touch with your inner strength, courage, wisdom, patience, determination, self-love, and compassion, you can create permanent change.

Exercise 9: Bringing in Your Divine Qualities

Because you've been out of touch with yourself and the wonderful qualities you possess, you've been looking outside yourself for validation and identity. The real truth of your being is that you're made up of many beautiful qualities that emanate from your soul. These are Divine talents given to you by your Creator. When you invoke the Highest Presence within yourself by remembering the name of the Most High in your heart, you can start to perceive these attributes that are your essence. As you reacquaint yourself with them and reabsorb them into the very fiber of your being, they'll slowly start to be reflected in your life more and more.

AS GOD SEES YOU

You could spend a lot of time bolstering your ego, trying to convince yourself that you're a good person or that you don't really eat more than someone who's thin, but that judgment can always be challenged. Instead, why not move beyond the limitations of your mind-body-personality to the part of you that is and always will be perfect—your true, Divine nature?

The more you identify with your essence in this way, the more likely you are to begin acting it out in your life. Your self-image will naturally begin to change as you let go of your past perceptions. You'll no longer have to be the person who hates exercise and feels like it's disgusting and unsophisticated to sweat. You'll be free of your identity as having absolutely no willpower and needing to reward yourself with a bag of chips when you get home from work.

Why not cultivate a closer relationship with the part of you that's eternal rather than spending a lifetime trying in vain to fix what you perceive to be broken? When you choose the former, the limited identities will simply melt away. You'll develop a true knowing that those perceptions were fabricated over time and can be released.

The best way to discharge your old, outdated, and hurtful self-image is to go deep inside and see yourself as God does. You can do this by learning to use the "eye of your heart," rather than your critical mind. For instance, you may have a lot of evidence that you're uptight or anxious and can't get through the day without caffeine or chocolate. Well, even if everyone you know confirms this, it doesn't make that perception correct. The ultimate truth is that Divine peace and calm is your true nature, and you could stop drinking coffee and eating candy in a minute—even if you aren't yet experiencing this aspect of yourself, or expressing it in the world.

Sometimes you may forget that your Creator is absolutely compassionate and merciful. The qualities of your Source are the ones within you. How many times have you berated yourself for eating too much? Do you ever gaze in the mirror and acknowledge your inner beauty, or do you simply cringe when you look at the fat on your body?

It's only by learning to receive attributes such as compassion and mercy that you can start to give to yourself—and to the world—in a very important way. When you receive compassion from the infinite supply of the Universe you become filled with it, so much so that the caring naturally starts running over, like a cup of water that's been spilling over the brim. The more that you're able to look in the mirror and see your beauty and essential goodness and give yourself compassion, the less you'll feel the need to nurture yourself with food.

After bingeing on meals that make you feel like a pig, the last thing you need to add insult to injury is hurtful comments from yourself about how disgusting you are. Instead, a little mercy may prompt you to really find ways to change your lifestyle and eating habits for good. You need to open up and receive love and compassion for yourself so that it can help you stay in alignment with your goal and ultimately flow into the world around you.

I like the expression "If you want to be generous, it's good to be rich." In other words, you can have an abundance of any quality when you receive it from the infinite supply of the Source.

THE QUALITIES THAT TRANSFORM YOU

When you ask God to change your perceptions, you'll begin to witness yourself and others as God does. It's as if you're asking for a second opinion: "I see that I am fearful, God, but how do *You* see me?" By calling in the higher qualities of your deeper self, you'll start to witness these aspects in your life more and more. This is important so that you can stop relating to yourself in such a limited and unproductive way.

Here are some things to keep in mind about some wonderful attributes that you have:

— You may not experience yourself as having any **patience** at all. It may feel downright frustrating to have to start at square one with exercise when you're so out of shape and overweight. However, when you call on the Divine quality of patience, you'll start to discover that there's a universal supply of this virtue that you can tap in to in order to transform your experience of working out.

— One of my favorite things to work with and draw into my heart is **holiness**. When you invoke this, you can start to experience yourself beyond any obsessions with food or counterproductive yo-yo dieting. Instead, you can connect to a sacred place inside yourself, which in the past you may have felt separate from. As you begin to experience a greater sense of godliness inside, you'll start to treat yourself differently. All of a sudden you may find yourself wanting to eat water-rich foods to support a healthy body, mind, and spirit, because you're in touch with how sacred and special your life really is.

— You can also work with **awareness,** since you may be unaware of the unconscious eating behaviors you regularly indulge in. Maybe you're at the refrigerator all night long without any conscious thought. When you begin to bring in the attribute of Divine awareness, this invocation becomes like a prayer to help you become more mindful of your behaviors so that you can stop the automatic programs that are harmful to you.

— So often you may eat as a way to calm yourself. When you work with the quality of **peace,** however, and really draw it into your heart and soul, you'll return to a state of inner calm. Not only can you have harmony in any moment, but you can tap in to an infinite supply from your Creator.

— **Safety** and **protection** are two blessings that can release you from a vague feeling of fear about your life to an inner knowing that you're resting in the unity of the Universal Life Force. When this changes from a concept in your mind to an actual experience in your body through the following activity, you'll notice a profound shift in your relationship with food. When you feel comfortable in your own skin—and that you belong here and have the complete protection of your Maker—you'll begin to make selections that nourish and sustain you.

All of the qualities that you'll be working with are resources that can help you achieve the life you long for. These have always been inside you, but when you make a decision to access them, you'll notice a huge difference in your ability to stick to your goals.

In this exercise, you'll practice getting in touch with the higher qualities that you may well have forgotten you possess. I've written this to help you access the patience and compassion, but feel free to tailor it to any wonderful qualities that might help you in transforming your feelings, thoughts, and behaviors: Wisdom, strength, power, awareness, light, peace, safety, protection, truth, aliveness, creativity, mercy, generosity, holiness, openness, and gratitude are just a few that you might want to tap in to. You may want to work with one, two, or even three when you do this activity.

Record This Exercise

Take a few deep breaths and let your muscles relax as much as possible. Let your chair or sofa hold you up, allowing gravity to do its job. Feel your muscles go loose and limp, like a rag doll.

Begin the Remembrance exercise with the word or phrase for your Creator. Remember to allow the name to actually emanate from your heart center, as if you could see, feel, and even hear it there as you whisper it. With each repetition, allow the name to drop deeper into your core. Put your hand on your chest for a few moments to really connect with yourself. Consciously drop your awareness down into your heart and call in the higher vibration of light that's symbolized by the name of God. . . .

If you have trouble getting from your head to your heart, imagine something beautiful and peaceful in your center, like a rose, waterfall, or dew-covered meadow.

Now, bring in the quality of patience. You can draw it up from the deepest place in your heart and make it infuse all the layers of your being. Go slow and easy. Say the name of God as you inhale, and take the time to feel the vibration go through you. As you exhale, say, "Patience." Take it nice and slow. Inhale: "The One . . ." Exhale: "Patience . . ." Inhale: "Dear God . . ." Exhale: "Patience . . ."

Feel the patience within you. You can even see the word written in bright light deep within your heart.

Next, bring in the quality of compassion. Breathe the word and its essence in and out of your soul. Feel the softness and gentleness of this quality. . . . Inhale: "Compassion . . ." Exhale: "Divine compassion . . ."

Drink in the essence of this attribute deep inside. . . . You're floating on a sea of compassion. . . . This help is here for you now, for all your struggles . . . for all your hardships. Place your burdens down and allow yourself to swim in the ocean of absolute compassion. . . .

Doing this exercise—even for just ten minutes—will help you reduce anxiety and achieve a sense of inner calm and tranquility. If you can, continue for up to 30 minutes, each time drinking in the essence of the quality and the higher light emanating from it. Open yourself up to receive the blessing of patience, compassion, or whatever you're working with. Feel it seeping into your being.

By working with any of the Divine traits, it's as if you're planting the seed of that virtue and watering it with your intention, breath, and repetition.

A Commitment to Turning on the Light

Accessing your inner Source means choosing the voice of love over the voice of fear. It means making a decision to cherish yourself enough to break through the false identity you hold of being out of control around food or only desiring unhealthy things. As you face challenges, you'll have to renew this commitment over and over again. But when you follow through on your decision to choose love, you'll start to become aware of all the beautiful ways in which your life is shifting. This will give you the impetus to persevere toward your goal, no matter how compelling or real fear appears to be in your life. It only stays dark until you turn on the light. There is, in fact, no other way to dispel the gloom.

When you turn to your Creator with deep sincerity, you're turning on that light. You're affirming that you choose love, even if the outer evidence delivered to you from your five senses disputes that this God even exists. You can make this choice over and over again, despite the voices that may be screaming in your head, "You're being conned! Look at you—you'll always be overweight! Food is your greatest pleasure—there's nothing else that will satisfy you!" Every time you turn away from those fears, you're rewarded with an even deeper connection to the Source of love and a strengthening of your inner knowing that change is not only possible, it's happening for you.

You can't always convince your mind to take a backseat to your heart. But the more you take that leap of faith, the easier it will become. You'll get to a point where you realize with humility and gratitude that this is the way you were always meant to live.

The only way to truly understand how empowering and enriching this connection is, is to make it. What have you got to lose? Experiment with letting your heart take the lead, with asking for help and answers from your own inner wisdom, with taking the time to wash clean the voices that no longer serve you in the next few steps, and see how your life transforms.

CHAPTER SEVEN

Step 3: Accept Yourself as You Are

One of the crucial steps to successful weight loss is accepting yourself just as you are today—no matter what your mental, physical, or emotional state is. It can be very challenging to do this, especially if you're not happy with what you're experiencing. You may ask, "How can I accept that I binge regularly, hardly exercise, am 25 pounds overweight, and have completely let myself go?"

However, until you make peace with yourself and your current condition, you're powerless to change. Until you say yes to what your life experience is right now, you'll continually find yourself in a state of conflict, wanting things to be different. How can you be in harmony if you're at war within, hurting yourself with your thoughts and behaviors? How can you effect lasting change in your life if you're spending so much energy hating and judging yourself?

Do you believe that you and the people around you need to be perfect in order for you to be happy? The beauty and harmony that you seek in the outer world is actually within you. When you accept all aspects of yourself, you'll discover that this includes the part of you that wants to "pig out" at lunchtime or that seeks fulfillment through food.

If you can't come to terms with (and give love and redirection to) the parts of you that aren't currently on board with your goal, you're going to hit a wall of frustration or emptiness over and over. Like a child clamoring for his mother's attention, any part of you that you reject can take on a life of its own and act out in very destructive ways, such as out-of-control eating.

We all tend to separate and judge parts of ourselves, creating an inner environment of separation and angst. Well, you can choose to stop doing this, even if it feels unfamiliar to be at peace inside. Be merciful and love yourself, even as you're perceiving your weaknesses.

All too often, you may forget to have compassion for your own humanity and the difficulties and challenges you face. Even if you feel disconnected from your sense of kindness and are much more in touch with cynicism and judgment, you still have the capacity to return to your true, innate attribute of love.

When you're forgiving toward yourself, it doesn't mean that you condone actions that hurt you or sabotage your plans. You won't say, "Oh well, I binge on an entire bag of chips almost every night and that's okay, so I'm not going to do anything about it." What you'll do is stop spending time beating yourself up and instead focus your energy on looking at some of your motivations, discovering where you're going wrong, and figuring out strategies that can help you fulfill your own needs and achieve your heart's true desire.

You may think that if you're hard enough on yourself, you can force yourself to change. In fact, the opposite is true: Berating yourself gets you feeling so miserable that you give up any motivation to persevere toward your goals. When you truly honor and accept yourself exactly as you are right now, however, it's much easier to transform your thoughts and behaviors.

Understanding Your Inner Child

If your inner climate is one of self-judgment and harsh feelings toward yourself, how will you ever find the energy, courage, and optimism to attempt to change? You need to know that you're worthy of the effort and that you absolutely can succeed. You aren't your mental programs or the resulting behaviors—they're simply veils keeping you from experiencing the deeper truth of who you are.

Positive reinforcement is so much more effective than punishment. Do you beat your pet until it does what you want? Of course not! You reward it, giving it love so that it naturally wants to please you. Most modern-day parenting books will tell you that the best way to raise happy, productive children is with positive reinforcement and natural consequences to behavior—not punishment. Your inner child needs the exact same thing from you. She's causing you to overeat not because she's bad and intends to hurt you, but because she cares about you and mistakenly thinks that there's a benefit to your indulging in food. Your inner child finds comfort in the meals and has found that consuming more is a way to avoid painful feelings such as insecurity, hurt, or worry.

Of course your inner child wants to protect you and bring you pleasure—to that end, she encourages you to enjoy what tastes good, regardless of whether it's healthy for you. She also reminds you that exercise makes your muscles ache; since you don't want to feel bad, you listen to her guidance and avoid working out.

Although this part of you really only wants you to experience pleasure, she doesn't understand what's happening as a result of this childish behavior. When the inevitable anguish and shame of your habits surface, you turn on yourself with blame, disgust, and hurtful self-talk. Then when you berate yourself this way, your inner child gets wounded and becomes even more determined to avoid pain and seek pleasure. And the vicious circle goes 'round and 'round.

However, when you stop being hard on yourself and simply accept your current state and what's actually happening, you're much more likely to engage in behaviors that will support you and lead to achieving your vision.

Help Your Inner Child Find a New Way

Your vulnerable but often-misguided inner child is one part of yourself that you must come to terms with if you want to transform your behaviors. Acknowledge and thank her for looking out for your interests, but let her know that she needs to revise her ideas about what will serve you.

If you can show your needy inner child a much more positive way to get her needs met, you may be surprised to find that she'll follow your lead and do what you want. She simply needs to be updated on the natural consequences of her behavior, since these have changed over time.

If you look to the past, these unhealthy eating behaviors served you when you initially began them. The food did taste good, and you experienced pleasure while consuming it—there's no denying that. But perhaps you've never stopped to consider that antifreeze might taste good, too. I'm sure you'd never knowingly drink that substance, even if you'd been told it was absolutely delicious, because you've accepted that it's poison. The benefit of experiencing a pleasant taste sensation would not outweigh the dire consequences.

But if someone offered you a rich, sugary, empty-calorie, fat-laden dessert—which is equally poisonous to your system in the long run—you'd very likely dig in, simply because you want pleasure . . . and your inner child is more than happy to give it to you. You've tricked your mind into associating joy with even the most poisonous substances because society condones it, an attractive or friendly person is serving it, it comes wrapped up in a very nice package, or advertising encourages you to indulge in it. At that moment, your inner child has no concept of how short-lived the pleasure is and the huge price that you're paying by setting yourself up for chronic food addiction.

It's time to stop blaming your inner child for these harmful behaviors, and instead, love her, accept her, and teach her a new way to be. As you continue on the six steps to permanent weight loss, you'll be able to help her find a better way to achieve the love, safety, and happiness she's seeking. The more she fulfills these needs, the less she'll have to turn to food to satisfy the insatiable need for nurturing and love.

Exercise 10: Accepting What Is

You may have an idea of how you want yourself and your life to be. Unfortunately, this most likely doesn't correspond to the way things actually are. What's happening is that you're resisting what is. Anytime you do this, you're going to suffer. You may assume that it's the event that's causing you pain, but it isn't—it's your *resistance* to the event. The next time you say or do something that you wish you hadn't, feel the regret and just say yes to it. You may be tempted to make up a story about it and rationalize, judge, or analyze what happened; instead, just say yes.

Record This Exercise

Close your eyes and get comfortable. Notice how you're feeling right now: Are you holding tension in your jaw, your pelvic region, or anywhere else in your body? Observe your breathing: Is it deep or shallow? Don't think about how you're supposed to be breathing. Simply notice what your experience is in this moment.

Think about the current situation with your weight. Bring to mind your bigger story of being heavy—its causes, history, effects, and impact on your life. Let yourself witness all of the emotions involved. Perhaps you feel helplessness, guilt, anger, frustration, embarrassment, or pain. Allow yourself to stay with this entire scenario and everything associated with it, without trying to change, fix, or rationalize it. Accept what is. Don't give in to the urge to distract yourself, make a joke, come up with a solution, downplay it, cope with it, or stop this exercise altogether.

Feel your resistance, and let yourself be okay with it, without acting on it or trying to get rid of it. Be willing to be uncomfortable if that's how you feel. Realize that the discomfort stems from your reluctance to be with what is, not the outer circumstances. It's through feeling the feelings that you can achieve a breakthrough.

Next, imagine that you can see yourself in front of you, as if you're looking in the mirror. Look at yourself with the eyes of compassion, not judgment, and just say yes. Say yes to you . . . to all of you . . . to the parts that you like . . . and the ones that you don't. Say, "I accept you fully."

Approve of yourself in the fullness of who you are in this moment. You aren't your behavior or fears. Tell yourself, "I would prefer it if you did/didn't do _____, but I accept you fully in your state of _____." If there's any judgment in your words, tone, or thoughts, let that be okay, too. Say, "I accept that I judge myself as ____ _____."

Remember that your emotions aren't good or bad; they just are. Your state of mind is like the weather: constantly changing. You don't have to act on every feeling that flows through you, because it's simply energy in motion. Allow yourself to be, without censoring.

If you're feeling a strong emotion, ask yourself, *Why am I feeling this? What belief or picture am I holding to be true?* See if you can discover and sit with whatever is behind the sensation.

As you gaze at your image in the "mirror," begin to witness yourself without judgment. There's some part of your consciousness that's always in this watching mode. Simply shift your awareness to identify with this aspect of yourself, as opposed to your ego.

Take one last look and imagine yourself as you were when you were just being born, emerging into the world. Visualize this baby that you were, coming into your adult arms. How do you feel about yourself now? Witness yourself holding this beautiful soul that you are as a baby in your own arms. Take your time.

When you're ready, come back into the room.

The Effects of Stress

One of the main difficulties in accepting yourself exactly as you are may be that you overeat because you're feeling stressed out and can't seem to stop yourself. Again, be compassionate. You probably underestimate just how stressful your life is, and you haven't been taught healthy ways to manage the high levels of stress you deal with in this fast-paced world. It's only natural that you try to soothe and comfort yourself when you're feeling frazzled. If you can understand where the stress is coming from and find better ways to manage it, your inner child won't pressure you to curl up in a big comfortable chair and overeat.

Aside from the emotional and physical strain of being overweight, the tensions of life have an impact on all your bodily systems, whether you like it or not. You might not realize it, but physical ailments such as migraines, gastrointestinal problems, backaches, knee pain, and acne may all clear up as if by magic when you start managing stress in a healthy way instead of reaching for unhealthy food as your medicine. And when you start increasing your activity level (which is an excellent stress-buster), you may also experience sudden cures to physical problems that have plagued you for a long time.

The reality is that you must learn to manage stress because, like everyone else, you're always going to have some kind of tension. It may be positive, such as starting a new job, or negative, such as dealing with a traffic jam—but your body instinctively reacts to *all* changes and challenges as if they were threatening. The automatic response that you were born with originally developed in order to help primitive humans survive, but it rarely serves that purpose anymore. This reflex—an increased heart rate, fast and shallow breathing, muscle contracting, blood vessels constricting, and the release of chemicals into your body—is triggered whether you're getting married or divorced, winning the lottery, or crashing your car.

In the past, you may have calmed these unpleasant effects with food. Today, you can learn to combat these side effects of life by using deep relaxation techniques that will reverse your body's response.

HIDDEN STRESSES

If you're thinking that stress isn't affecting your body because you haven't experienced a huge life change recently, remember that everyday problems can have a strong impact as well. Yours may come from the anxieties you create for yourself.

You probably spend a lot of time in your head—thinking, analyzing, and thinking some more. You wouldn't be reading this book if you didn't have intelligence that's helped you create success in many areas of your life. Your mind is a wonderful tool and there's nothing wrong with thinking, but it's easy to make the mistake of assuming that you are your mind. You get stuck in your head and leave your body behind, which causes tension, anxiety, and unwanted habits that you use as coping mechanisms and may ultimately lead to illness or disease. It's not that you should stop thinking, but you'll want to have your mind be in service to your heart, rather than taking the lead itself.

You may assume that you're being productive or figuring things out, but in reality you're more than likely spinning your wheels by replaying the same thoughts and pictures continually and worrying about them: what you ate for lunch, guilt over being too short-tempered with your spouse this morning, how you look in your clothes, and so on. This mental whirlwind is having a very detrimental effect on your body, even if you aren't aware of it. You may be tightening your muscles, particularly in your jaw, face, neck, shoulders, back, belly, and pelvis.

Obsessive thinking can lead to high blood pressure and heart conditions, and it can certainly contribute to tension, anxiety, headaches, digestive disorders (such as irritable bowel syndrome), overeating, bingeing, snacking, and emotional eating. Of course all of these health conditions make you depressed, unmotivated to change your life, tired, and reluctant to exercise. So to distract yourself from the emotional and physical aches and pains, you may well turn to food.

Do you feel your body constricting when circumstances aren't to your liking? If you're not sure, check in with your belly. This is where many of us hold tension, fear, or nervousness. Your abdominal area is where your inner child energetically resides—it's the part of you that may feel abandoned, rejected, insecure, or afraid. When many people get upset, they feel their stomach "tied up in knots" or contracted. There are many nerve connections between the brain and the gut, so this isn't just a metaphor—there's a physiological connection that causes this stress reaction.

As the demands on you increase—from your spouse, children, extended family, work, body, friends, and other obligations—you may not know where to turn to summon the energy you need. If you're like most of my clients, it can be challenging for you to cope with the multitude of requests for your time. You may have created a life for yourself that includes everything you want—career, family, success, friendships, and community—but even so, you're juggling so many balls that you wonder how long it will be before you drop one. Unprepared for the obvious (and hidden) stresses you face, you can easily fall into stress eating.

STRESS EATING

You may feel that you need to use food to make you feel more in control of a stressful situation: "If I'm going to have to work late again tonight, then I'm going to treat myself to a big, juicy cheeseburger for dinner." Or you may be bored or depressed because you don't have enough activity in your life (not enough stimulation is also a form of stress), so you use food as a way to comfort and energize yourself: "I'm bored. Maybe I'll whip up a batch of brownies and enjoy them."

Accept that tension is an inevitable part of life and that you'll always be challenged to manage it. If you aren't good at doing so, that's okay; the following exercises are going to teach you healthy methods. If you continue to let stress control your life, you'll pay the price of being overweight, anxious, tired, dissatisfied, and at risk for a multitude of disorders.

But as you learn stress-management techniques, you'll get healthier and use rest, deep breathing, and physical activity to help you naturally increase your energy or relax yourself. You'll no longer rely on food as a tool for managing anxiety, and you'll soon become free of those toxic side effects—and you can do this at any age!

You'll start to live at a more comfortable pace and feel like you're in greater control of your body, mind, and eating habits. Even with the ups and downs of life, you can naturally begin to exist from a more peaceful place. This will lead to your making decisions and setting priorities based on your heartfelt longings, rather than the whims and influences of your environment.

SOME SIMPLE STRESS-BUSTING TECHNIQUES TO USE EVERY DAY

It's important to develop emergency strategies for moments of frustration or weakness. When you feel your body tensing up and a knot forming in your stomach, take a breath and realize that you're beginning to have a physiological response to stress. Make a decision to stay conscious of your reaction, remain connected to yourself, and relax in your body as best you can in spite of the circumstances. In the middle of picking up your kids, reading an upsetting memo from your boss, or making dinner, you can always take a deep breath and let it out, making the "Aaaah" sound with each exhalation. And with your eyes open or closed, you can visualize a brilliant light in your heart center.

You might also say to yourself, *I don't like these circumstances. I would prefer it if I wasn't running 15 minutes late to this appointment, but the traffic is here. That's just the way it is. This isn't in my control, and I accept it as it is.* Of course, you may wish that you had anticipated this scenario and left earlier, and maybe next time you'll do that. But rather than hammer yourself with criticism, take a deep breath and realize that in this moment you're learning a lesson, as painful as it may be.

It can also be helpful to remind yourself that even if you'd left a half hour earlier, you could have been deterred by an accident or any act of nature. So be gentle with yourself, and take the opportunity to be present and learn.

You can silently ask to be shown a deeper reality when things in your immediate environment seem out of control. In the privacy of your own mind, you can say to your Creator, *Right now I'm in chaos,*

*my body feels tight all over, and the voices in my head are screaming,
"Go get a candy bar!" Please help me. Show me how to see the situation
with Your eyes and with Your ears. Help me act in a way that's in alignment with the bigger picture of my life and my true essence, and not my
wounded inner child. Thank You so much! I surrender to Your wisdom.*
Then just experience your inner guidance even as you're tending to
the outer world.

And if you find yourself reaching for food in moments of stress,
stop, close your eyes (if you can), and take two or three deep breaths.
Mentally affirm: *I accept everything exactly as it is. I don't prefer it, but
it's not my choice. I say yes to my life.* Place your hand on your heart or
on your belly and consciously send yourself some love and mercy.

REDUCING STRESS THROUGH AWARENESS

To begin to reduce your stress level—even in this moment as
you're reading—you can become more in touch with your physical body and what you're feeling right now. It helps to notice your
breath, no matter what's happening in your environment. When you
start to breathe more fully and deeply in each moment, your stress
level will begin to subside.

By expanding your awareness, you aren't simply telling yourself
to relax; you're calming down naturally. When someone tells you to
relax, you may find yourself doing the opposite. However, if you simply open your awareness to include your breathing and the sensations
in your entire body, relaxation spontaneously occurs.

When you open your consciousness, your entire perspective will
shift from a small, narrowly focused, limited viewpoint within your
head to a wider, all-encompassing experience of expansion through
your body. It will become easier to tune out the external distractions
and tune in to the world of your soul. When you do, you'll feel yourself in the depths of the ocean of life rather than tossed about on its
turbulent waves. You'll learn to notice the aspect of yourself that's a
silent, nonjudgmental witness—the you who simply watches as you
think, feel, and move through the day.

As you begin to discover this inner observer and your stress level decreases, you'll feel a new freedom wash over you. The more you can accept whatever you're experiencing, the more you'll be able to let go and melt into the greater reality at the core of your being, well beyond whatever's happening in the outer world. Now, the choices that you'll begin to make and the actions that result will truly support your mind, body, and spirit.

The more you cultivate your ability to simply witness yourself, the less you'll judge yourself or get caught up in the stresses of the day that in the past would have triggered negative eating behaviors. For example, in the past if you had a difficult day at work, you may have felt so upset that you went home, ate 2,000 calories, and then started hating yourself for it. When you identify less with the events of the day and your reaction to them, you may begin to spontaneously feel compassion for yourself and your situation. This is likely to lead you to the decision that you'll go swimming or play racquetball after work to burn off steam, instead of giving in to the old emotional eating.

When you let go of judgment, you'll begin to simply take notice of what's occurring. Even if you do react, you'll be able to just note it as it's happening. For example, let's say that you impulsively reach for the last piece of pie in the refrigerator. As you witness yourself pulling it out of the fridge, you'll be able to notice yourself and what you're thinking and feeling. *I really shouldn't be eating this—I'm already so fat,* one voice in your head might declare. Another voice may pipe in just as quickly, *Oh, come on . . . why not? You only live once—and besides, your weight isn't going anywhere. You'll always be fat.* Inside, you're likely to feel guilty and torn apart by the voices that are screaming in your head.

Witnessing the scenario as it's occurring in this way will give you an opportunity to gain some distance from this internal tug of war. Then, like a loving parent refereeing a squabble between two siblings, you'll be able to determine what's needed. It might be nothing more than sitting down and taking a few deep breaths . . . or reaching for some celery to hold you over . . . or drinking a full glass of water with apple-cider vinegar to cut cravings. New possibilities will open to you automatically.

So whenever you experience an uncomfortable feeling that gives you the impulse to act in a way that isn't in alignment with your vision, just watch it with curiosity, as if you were a scientist. Stop yourself from resisting or repressing what you're experiencing. If you're reaching for a piece of pie, for example, surrender to this reality and the feeling you have. Realize that whatever your thought, feeling, or impulse is, you're bigger than it is.

When you shift to the witness mode, your behavior goes from being completely unconscious to conscious. This is great news, because you're unlikely to hurt yourself consciously! By making yourself aware, you've pulled yourself out of the dissociated state that automatically engages in harmful behavior over and over again—now you can make a choice. Because you created your vision in Step 1 and began regularly connecting to your Source in Step 2, making a good choice will be much easier than it ever was before.

Exercise 11: Cultivating the Inner Witness

You don't need to record this exercise—simply read it once or twice and go through it in your mind:

Think of a scenario in your life right now that's troubling you—a person or situation that you feel is robbing you of your happiness. You may have a belief that if this one particular person or problem were different, everything would be fine.

Imagine this painful scenario now, and as you do, begin to shrink the image down. Watch it become smaller . . . smaller, so tiny that you can hold the picture of the problem in your left hand. . . . If there's any sound to the scenario (such as a person's voice), imagine it coming from your left hand.

As you listen to this voice coming from your left hand, create a grounding cord that reaches from the center of your belly all the way to the hot, molten core of the earth; make it strong and thick. Feel your roots coming down from your legs and planting themselves deep into the ground.

Next, see in your mind's eye a beautiful, tall tree. Perhaps it's a huge old banyan or oak, standing strong and powerful. Bring this feeling into your body. Lean against the tree and drink in its ever-present strength.

As you hold the image of your problem in your left hand, notice how different it seems. Now you're witnessing it.

When you're ready, open your eyes and come back into the room.

You can do the above exercise with any emotion, judgment, or situation. You no longer need to be the victim of your environment. Instead of feeling drained or pulled, as you witness your experiences—rather than being sucked in by them—you'll be able to more easily focus on what you're here to give. In that moment, it may be nothing more than to radiate the peace that's at the core of your being.

ACCEPTANCE IS A PROCESS

Accepting yourself doesn't require you to resolve all your issues. After all, each cloud is only a small part of the vast sky, and even when one completely hides the sun, inevitably it will pass. The sun never loses its radiance, even when the sky is filled with thunderheads. Your unfavorable feelings about yourself are like this, and the light that you bring into this world is incomparable and undeniable, no matter how disconnected you feel from it in the moment.

The more you cultivate the witness aspect of yourself, the greater a resource it becomes. It's much easier to accept yourself fully when you identify with your ego less, and more so with the silent observer that's an inherent part of you. It simply takes practice. At first, it may take a lot of effort to remember to observe yourself. The more you practice the technique in Exercise 11, the more it will become second nature, similar to riding a bicycle or tying your shoes. At one time, you probably thought that you'd never master such difficult tasks. But all it takes is practice, commitment, and an understanding of the value of this skill. Being the witness helps you say yes to what is, be less easily upset by your surroundings, accept whatever's happening in the moment, and stay centered in your body.

Exercise 12: Expanding Your Awareness

Practicing this lesson regularly will help remind you to change your focus from a limited viewpoint to that of a broader reality that inherently carries the solutions you seek.

It's helpful to attempt this particular awareness exercise with your eyes both open and closed. Normally, when you close your eyes while doing any of the relaxation and centering techniques, you can have a fuller experience. However, when you do this one with your eyes open, it makes it easier to transition the stress reduction into daily life, giving you greater benefits.

The point of this activity isn't to take 20 minutes, center yourself fully, get deeply relaxed, and then move back into your life at full throttle, quickly eliminating the benefits. Rather, the goal is to slowly change your way of relating to your internal and external environment. Therefore, after you've done it a few times with your eyes closed, open-eyed practice can be of great benefit.

Record This Exercise

In a quiet space, get yourself situated comfortably and become aware of your breathing. Stay with your breath for several inhalations and exhalations. Notice the rhythm and your body's simultaneous movement. Enjoy all the sensations: Feel your skin and the temperature of the air in the room against your body.

If your eyes are closed, then see the objects around you in your mind's eye, and also notice the space around them and all that's in the periphery. Take your time. . . .

Can you hear any sounds in the background? Listen . . . is there the hum of an air conditioner or noise from traffic? Can you hear your own breathing? Notice the silence behind these noises, the peace out of which they emerge and that they fall back into.

Feel your face: Can you discern your mouth, including your lips, teeth, gums, and tongue? What does your jaw feel like?

Bring your awareness to your eyes and all the muscles in and around them. Feel that space between your eyebrows and your hairline. How does that area of your body feel? Are you holding any tension there? Focus on your scalp, and then your entire head. Imagine that you can feel inside your ears, nose, and skull. Open your awareness to this space.

Become aware of your hands. Take your time and feel the space in and around each finger. Are there any sensations in them or your fingertips?

Is the temperature hot or cold? Can you feel your clothes against your skin? Contemplate for a moment that your whole body is filled with space. It permeates all of your organs, muscles, bones, and cells. . . . Understand what it's like to feel this. Focus on your skin and imagine that it's permeable. Believe that you can breathe through your skin. . . .

Be aware of the area all around you filling the whole room. Visualize the boundaries of your body dissolving and the inside and outside of you as one continuous being. See the expanse beyond the room that you're in, farther out than the building . . . the space that fills the whole city, state, and country that you're in . . . and on and on to eternity. . . .

Is there any part of your body that feels tight or contracted? Bring to mind a situation that causes you to overeat or that makes your belly contract, such as being criticized or having to deal with chaotic surroundings. Just allow yourself to accept what you're feeling. . . . It's okay to experience discomfort. Go with your reaction to this situation without judging yourself in any way. Stay with that emotion, whatever it is. . . . Surrender to it completely.

Notice that your mental state has a physical component, and move closer to the strongest sensation in your body. . . . What are you feeling? Scan from the top of your head to the tips of your toes and find the part that's clamoring for your attention. Can you describe the sensation to yourself? If it had a color, what would it be? Is there a size or a shape to it?

Now, let this area of your body dissolve into the greater space that you occupy, and all the space beyond it. Allow the boundaries of the constricted area to dissolve and merge with everything around you.

Whenever you're ready, come back into the room. Take a moment to shake out your hands and feet.

EXPANDING AWARENESS THROUGHOUT THE DAY

Throughout the day, check in with yourself to determine what your level of awareness is. Don't beat yourself up if you discover that you've been lost in thought for the past hour. Simply redirect yourself in the moment. The easiest place to start is your breathing: To remind yourself to do this, you can place little stickers that say "Breathe" around your house, or you can tell yourself that every time the phone rings you'll check your awareness. It can also be helpful to get a watch with an alarm that goes off hourly. When you hear it, ask yourself, *How's my focus? Am I grounded? Am I feeling my feet firmly planted on the ground? How is my breathing—deep or shallow?*

See if your mind is open or contracted. Notice whether your thoughts are positive or negative. Are you aware of the silence between them, and can you expand this space consciously? Where does the idea go when you move on to the next one? Where does it come from when it returns? Tune in to the gap.

As you begin to notice your physical and emotional state through-out the day without judgment or criticism, you'll become aware of your impulses to grab a candy bar before you actually do it. Your new level of awareness, coupled with your commitment to change, will transform these old impulses naturally and lead you to healthier actions, such as eating an apple instead.

If you live in your head, detached from your physical self and unaware of the tight muscles or gurgling in your stomach, it might be because you're so unhappy with your body that you don't honor and nurture it. When you feel these aches and pains, pay attention. Don't tell yourself, *Oh, there goes my gut, gurgling again . . . what-ever. I always have stomach problems—that's just me. It's embarrassing. It's probably because I'm fat. That's an uncomfortable thought. I'm not going to deal with that. Where's the Maalox to stop this so that I don't have to think about my messed-up gut and being fat?* It's far better to be aware of that sensation and use your food diary and your inner wisdom to discover what's causing it and how you can stop it.

Be aware of your body, your feelings, and your thoughts. Remem-ber, as soon as you say yes to your current set of circumstances—even though you don't prefer them, your body will relax because there won't be any more struggle. You'll still be very aware of the impact of what's occurring, but you won't be at the mercy of it. You'll be able to make a conscious choice about what to do next based on the result that you want.

For example, perhaps your current set of circumstances is that you have to make a speech next week, and you've recently gained ten more pounds! You're feeling embarrassed and dread having to face your peers at your current weight. When you fully accept the situation as it is—that you're going to give the presentation, you're currently 30 pounds overweight, and you're freaking out about it—you'll begin to become aware of a greater perspective. You'll realize that you aren't the first heavy person to stand up in front of other people, and that what's really important isn't your weight but the material that you have to share. You can tune in to your excitement about that.

From this vantage point, you're also more likely to gain the insight necessary to make permanent shifts in your eating habits and lifestyle so that you aren't put in this situation again. The feeling of dread will dissolve, and you may begin to feel empowered, even though you would have preferred not to face this challenge. You may even be grateful for this set of circumstances as they finally provide you with the motivation that you need.

Practicing the exercises you've learned in Step 3 will help move you from the "I'm good or I'm bad" way of thinking to the more responsible mode of putting aside your tendency to judge or criticize yourself and instead tuning into your behaviors so that you can ask yourself, *What are the likely consequences of this behavior? Given that, what choice do I want to make at this time in order to achieve what my heart truly desires?*

As you learn to give yourself love and acceptance, even the most "resistant" parts of yourself—such as the part that still wants to eat whatever it wants, when it wants, with no planning ahead—will jump on board to help you achieve the vision that you hold for your life.

CHAPTER EIGHT

Step 4: Break Free from Obstacles

There's a place within you that's been there all along but that you probably haven't made contact with too often. The purpose of journeying to your heart is to get in touch with that part—your inner wisdom, which knows and wants what's best for you. Your guidance will show you new ways to respond to the challenges or situations that in the past have caused you to overeat, binge, snack, or engage in emotional eating.

Exercise 13: Contacting Your Inner Wisdom

You'll start this exercise by using your permanent-weight-loss journal to log your answers to important questions about the obstacles that are blocking you from shedding pounds. Then you'll do a guided meditation, which you should record.

In your journal, write down the answers to these questions about blocks to achieving and maintaining your ideal weight. Look at the triggers that cause you to reach for food. Do you:

- Eat when you're standing up?

- Snack while you're watching TV?

- Keep food in the car?

- Tend to serve yourself huge portions?

- Help yourself to seconds before you even finish what's in front of you?

- Go for long periods of time without eating, only to binge later?

- Eat when you aren't physically hungry?

- Use food to manage your moods—when you're angry, lonely, sad, and so on?

- Drink diet soda that seems to satisfy you, but which is actually exacerbating your overweight condition and sugar cravings?

- Finish everything on your plate even when you're already stuffed?

- Gobble so fast that you don't even realize when you're full?

- Snack when you're tired to boost your energy level or regulate your blood sugar?

- Overeat regularly when you're socializing?

- Have difficulty walking away when dessert is being served?

Record This Exercise

Take a few deep breaths and close your eyes. Ground yourself by sinking a cord from your center of power—that orange ball of fire just below your navel—down into the hot, molten core at the center of the earth. Feel your legs and imagine that they're roots traveling down into the soil, connecting you with the strength and power of this great planet. You're solid, like the greatest tree.

Get in touch with your metaphorical heart by gently resting your hand on your upper chest and breathing in and out underneath your hand. Feel fullness as you inhale and exhale. With each breath, allow your awareness to travel deeper into this area. Imagine two nostrils in the center of your heart, as if you were actually inhaling and exhaling from this point.

If you find yourself distracted with thoughts about your day, just come back to the physical sensation of your hand on your chest. Take your time breathing in . . . and out . . . feel the steadiness and the rhythm . . . cool air coming in, warm going out. With each exhalation, imagine that any tension leaves your body.

Continue to breathe in and out of your heart center. To help access this place more strongly, recall or imagine a situation when you felt very safe, protected, and connected with all of life. It could be when you were out in nature, alone or with a loved one; maybe you were witnessing a glorious sunrise or a beautiful garden. Perhaps it was a time of profound joy, such as your wedding or the day you gave birth to your baby, or a time when you were listening to wonderful music or creating art. See the bright and beautiful colors of this scene, hear any sounds, and feel all the pleasant sensations. Imagine this very peaceful time or place as you continue to breathe in and out of your heart center, traveling deeper with each breath.

Allow a word, phrase, or picture describing this experience to come to you. It could be a symbol of faith or something calling out to you from your own wisdom. Allow it to come to you; when it does, see it written in light across your chest. Take a moment and stay with this image as you feel all of the pleasant, soothing sensations.

Now bring to mind one of the obstacles that you wrote down earlier. Recall a situation that in the past would have caused you to engage in unproductive eating habits or be sedentary. Notice how your body reacts when confronted by that experience. Take a moment to observe how it feels to want to automatically binge, consume the wrong foods out of habit, feast when you aren't hungry, or eat for emotional reasons. . . .

Return now to the luminous word, phrase, or picture in your heart center, and as you do, notice how the negative scenario somehow seems different when you're centered in this place within yourself. Does the situation fade to black and white or move farther off into the distance?

If there's sound, perhaps the volume gets turned way down. Be aware of how it feels to stay with that icon written in light across your own heart. Bring the scene of the obstacle into your core, and at the same time, imagine that the symbol connecting you to your deeper wisdom is written in light right over this scenario—as if it were superimposed. Stay with your powerful image in the depths of your chest. Continue to repeat this word or phrase to yourself as you see and feel it connecting with the internal picture you hold of the obstacle.

Ask your inner wisdom, which resides in this place within you, to show you a new way to respond to that trigger. Ask, *What can I do in the face of this obstacle?*

You don't need to think of a response. Just stay with your word, phrase, symbol, or picture, and allow it to guide you. Take all the time you need, and sink into a place of not knowing the answer. Wait patiently, breathing in and out of your chest. Perhaps it will come in the form of words, a picture, a feeling, or an idea. It might be as simple as seeing yourself drinking more water, carrying around healthy snacks so that you don't get ravenously hungry, or having more direct communication about what your needs are in situations that set you off emotionally. There's so much wisdom inside of you—patiently, allow it to guide you now. . . .

Next, imagine yourself adopting the positive behavior that frees you from food addiction. See yourself engaging in this new activity as if you've done it a hundred times in the past . . . as if it were perfectly natural for you. Imagine that you're living your life slender, healthy, fit, and at your ideal weight.

As you're engaging in this new, positive behavior that's aligned with your goals for yourself, see the environment that would surround you. . . . Hear the sounds of that place and time. . . . Notice all of the soothing sensations, and listen to your inner dialogue supporting and congratulating you. Feel the pride, joy, and exhilaration of knowing that your thoughts and behaviors are changing. You're achieving your goals, and your dreams are manifesting! Take a moment to give thanks to this creative, wise place inside of you.

Set your intention to return to this place over and over again, deepening your connection with your own source of inner wisdom and knowledge.

When you're ready, take your time and slowly come back into the room.

WRITE DOWN YOUR INSIGHTS

As with all the exercises, make sure to write down your insights from this session as soon as possible. If you aren't certain whether you received any significant information, be open to the possibility that your inner wisdom will continue to speak with you, since you've opened the doorway. For now, just make note of any insight you did gain. Also, write down the word, phrase, symbol, or picture that you were shown. This is a doorway for you to enter into this place within your center over and over again.

YOUR INNER WISDOM IS ALWAYS THERE TO GUIDE YOU

The more you practice getting in touch with your inner wisdom in the above exercise, the more you'll be able to draw on that resource in your daily life. For example, when you're about to eat, you can go inside to your place of safety and protection and request that your inner wisdom guide you. Ask, *What would be my best food choice now, in this moment?* Because your needs do change day to day, it's so helpful to access new, current input from the Source that truly knows. Maybe in this moment, a sandwich would be perfect for you, because it will tide you over until your next meal.

The beauty of using this method is that it helps keep you from the rigidity of "dieting" or the dangers of eating anything placed in front of you that looks or smells good. The more you go inside to find which foods are best for you in this moment, the more you can come to rely on this technique as a gift from your Creator.

Remember that it may take time for you to gain clarity on this inner communication, particularly if it's new to you, so track your results. If you're certain that when you asked inside which food on the menu would be best for you, the tuna salad "lit up," so you went ahead with that selection, take note of how you feel after the meal. If you feel good and light, then this is confirmation that you "read" your answer correctly. Then the next time you're in a similar situation and you ask your inner guidance for an answer, you'll have a better idea of what to listen for.

If the communication comes in a completely different way—for example, you start tasting the particular food that you're asking about—simply notice this. If you act on the insight, and the results are quite different from your previous experience, you will have learned a very valuable lesson about your inner system. Perhaps when something "lights up" for you, this is your deep wisdom speaking; but when a taste pops into your mouth, it's a signal for you to breathe, go deeper, and ask again. The flavor may even be a signal that you have a need such as nurturing or self-love.

The more that you learn about yourself in this way, the more you'll be able to break old, harmful routines and replace them with behaviors that truly serve you. In the process, you'll also be learning to trust yourself and value the wisdom that you carry in your core.

Exercise 14: What Should I Eat?

This exercise will help you break free of the obstacle of not knowing what to eat and assist you in making the best possible choice for yourself in the moment. (You don't need to record this exercise.)

Throughout the day, whenever you're unsure if you should eat—or what to have—close your eyes and connect with the deep inner wisdom in your heart. To do this, shift your awareness to your breath, and/or place your hand on your upper chest. Bow your head slightly to help you really focus on your core. Then ask your Source: What would be the best choice for me in this moment?

The more you're able to let go of any urgency about the response and adopt an attitude of trust and patience, the more likely it is that you'll find the answers coming to you with ease.

You can use this technique in other areas of your life as well. When you lose something, such as your glasses or keys, rather than running around frantically looking for them, it can be very helpful to get quiet, put your hand on your upper chest, and let your inner wisdom show you where you left them. The information will come, but you do need to request it. The asking is such a small step, yet it's essential.

I'm still astounded at how I can be pondering something or fretting about it for quite a while, yet as soon as I remember to get quiet and pray about it, I'm often given answers (or at least a deep sense of peace about the issue) almost instantaneously. As you practice this method, you'll receive many benefits, such as reducing stress. Your life can truly be transformed.

Are Internal Voices Sabotaging Your Efforts?

Probably some of the greatest obstacles that have sabotaged your success are the pictures and voices that run through your mind, almost like your own private film. This is your constant internal dialogue, the incessant commentary that you're often barraged with:

- "I have no willpower."

- "At my age (or with my hormones), I'll never lose weight. What's the difference? I might as well eat what I want."

- "You only live once, so I might as well enjoy myself."

- "I'm not that heavy compared to so-and-so."

- "I'll start my diet tomorrow."

- "I've been good all week, so I'll just have one."

- "I already cheated on my diet, so I might as well forget it."

- "So-and-so can eat anything she wants and never gain a pound. It just doesn't seem fair."

Does this sound familiar? It probably does. But instead of acting unconsciously when you hear these voices, you can stop and ask yourself, *Where is this coming from? Is it speaking to me for my own highest good? Does this voice know and want what's best for me?* The answer is "Of course not." These are simply old tapes and outdated programming that have been around in your psyche for a long time. Once you become aware of them, you can stop listening. Fortunately, when you do, the voices become less insistent. With this program, you're learning to get in touch with and listen to your inner wisdom, the voice that *does* know and want what's best for you.

Sometimes the voices you hear aren't even your own. They could be your internalization of your parents, teachers, friends, spouse, or some authority figure; or perhaps they're collective opinions from your particular culture. If you don't question their validity, you may take it for granted that they're based on reality and shouldn't be challenged. They could be the sound of mass consciousness telling you, "Indulge in rich foods and enjoy life!" or "This is *the* diet to be on." It could be rebellion against authority that says, "No one's going to tell *me* what to do or how to eat. I've been eating fried food my whole life, and I'm not about to stop now." Or you could be hearing the collective views of any faction in society.

These voices may seem like they're speaking the truth, but that often isn't the case. You can challenge them by bringing them to your inner Source, as you'll do in the remainder of this chapter.

DISCOVERING THE TRUTH WITH A CAPITAL "T"

When you're experiencing inner voices that give you messages about yourself and your relationship to food and exercise, let the light of Truth examine the voice and show you what is actually True with a capital "T," meaning absolute Truth, as opposed to a fact that can be changed. That I have short hair is a fact that can be disputed. That there's a place of deep wisdom within is a Truth that can't be altered. It may be true right now that I can't do any exercise—but the deeper Truth could be that with prayer and some physical intervention, such as acupuncture, my muscle pain will diminish and I'll be able to ride a bicycle.

When you bring the voices to the Light of Truth, you can move beyond the facts in this moment to the unlimited possibilities that exist for you. You can guess probabilities based on the past, but if you stay open to receive from the vast potential within your heart, you can be shown possibilities that you never would have thought existed.

The tricky thing about voices and beliefs is that they're almost always confirmed by your outer experience. That's why it often takes a connection to your deepest Source of strength to break through them. In other words, if you hold a belief that you're unloved, you'll always have plenty of proof in your environment. You'll see that your friends don't return your calls, your husband has too many outside interests, your co-workers treat you poorly, and so on. Inevitably, your environment proves to you that your belief is justified. This then confirms your other deeper beliefs, such as "There's something wrong with me" or "There's something bad about them." Tragically, you can spend your entire life not realizing that these outer "confirmations" are simply mirrors for a wound that you need to heal. It's life's way of showing you what you need to look at in order to grow.

Your deeply held convictions have probably been with you for a very long time, and perhaps they served you originally—or so it seemed. If you adopted a belief that you *love* to eat, it's because at the time food brought you comfort and disconnected you from pain, and you didn't know any other way to achieve that goal. Your positive intention was to be happy and safe. Unfortunately, this is obviously limiting because it doesn't take into account the much greater pain of being overweight, addicted to food, out of control, and in a state of compromised health. Then this became reinforced because whenever you did overeat or consumed sugary, rich foods, you felt better initially, and that's what you tuned in to. Your brain can make whatever you put into it come true; at the same time, it blocks out all other stimuli that run counter to what you're reinforcing. This is why what you believe seems to be true.

Because most people thrive on consistency and the sense of safety it creates, even when circumstances are painful, you may continue to unconsciously cause the conditions necessary for the painful situations to recur. Even in the face of evidence that's contrary to your belief, you may find yourself clinging to it. Consciously, you know that the way you love to eat is unhealthy and harmful. You can look around and see that a positive relationship with food is possible and more desirable, yet you still cling to the thought that this belief is true for you. You convince yourself that somehow you're different—that you could never eat in moderation the way a thin person does. Your negative conviction has you brainwashed to believe that your life would be empty without an unhealthy, compulsive relationship with food.

GETTING RID OF OLD BELIEFS

The mind is a complex collection of images, voices, and impressions from the past. These all come together to form your beliefs, values, and judgments. Then, like a tape recorder, your mind replays what you've taken in and created along the way. These ideas have often become deeply embedded, because you're constantly reinforcing them.

Beliefs are confirmed when you have a positive expectation that something will occur, you set yourself up to make it happen, it does, and you think, *I told you so!* If you spend the day thinking that you'll hate eating a healthy meal instead of indulging in pepperoni pizza, you will. If you think a thought enough, an entire belief system is developed through repetition.

The good news is you can change what you hold to be true by drawing on your desire, faith, and positive beliefs. Rather than basing your assumptions on what happened in the past, you can choose new ones that support you. Rather than thinking it's inevitable that you'll consistently overeat or you're destined to be fat, you can have faith that health and fitness are not only possible for you, but the natural order for your life.

It's time to change the pictures locked in your mind that stand in the way of what you truly want. All of the beliefs and obstacles that you hold in your subconscious are simply images. This means that although they're very real for you, and are in fact dictating your behavior, they aren't solid or carved in stone . . . and they can be updated.

For example, I had a belief for many years that I was bad at sports, because I have memories of being ridiculed as a child when I attempted to be athletic. Later, I discovered that I'm actually a very good runner, and I love to hike. Now I have internal pictures of thoroughly enjoying myself as I jog, bike, or hike. I've also gained the confidence to try other sports that I never had the opportunity to play, such as tennis and baseball. When you change your internal representations, your outer experience changes as well.

Remember to focus on what you *do* want, not what you don't. You're an expert at creating beliefs, so make a commitment to yourself for the next 40 days to consciously choose what you're going to focus on. If an old thought pops back into your head, as will undoubtedly happen, just notice it and gently turn your mind back. See it for what it is: an old belief fighting for its life. Look at that outdated concept and tell it firmly, "I'm a conscious being. I choose what I think. From now on, my beliefs support my deep, heartfelt desire to be healthy physically, mentally, and emotionally."

This is so important, because even though your logical mind may know, for example, that it's not true that no matter what you eat, you still gain weight, at a deeper level, you really do believe the lies you tell yourself. If you didn't, you wouldn't be acting on them daily . . . and they wouldn't be creating your reality.

Even though changing beliefs takes time and effort, it's well worth it. The Right Weigh program is helping you challenge your own self-talk until it matches your innermost desire to achieve permanent slenderness and be free from addiction.

THE POWER OF AWARENESS

The first step in discarding obstacles is to become aware of each one and its effect on your life. After that, you can no longer continue with those that are harmful. You can only keep engaging in things that are destructive to you if you're doing so unconsciously. How can you make your negative behaviors conscious? By setting your intention to open your awareness to the vicious cycle of negative beliefs that lead you to unhealthy behaviors.

Until you challenge these ideas, and ultimately transform them, your life is going to be dictated and controlled by these preexisting wounds and their current manifestations in your world. If you simply try to handle the outer situations—by going on a diet, getting divorced, moving to a different city, meeting new friends, or changing your job—you're going to continue to re-create the same or similar sets of circumstances.

Why not let your inner wisdom show you what's really true? You have the courage to let go of those voices and beliefs that no longer support you, even if you aren't in touch with it. The fact that you're reading this book and have a high level of desire confirms it. This program helps put you in touch with the option to stay connected to the highest voice of love that does, in fact, know and want what's best for you.

THE PROCESS OF BREAKING THROUGH YOUR OBSTACLES

Many times, the pictures in your head are beyond your conscious awareness. You may assume that the scenes floating through your mind are the only reality possible.

For example, I might have a fantasy about how wonderful it would be to sit down and eat a piece of chocolate cake. I might imagine how good it would taste and smell, how satisfying it would feel, and how relaxing it would be to sit and eat it. Rather than acting on this picture immediately, I'm able to stop and examine it. I can realize that yes, there's truth to this picture or belief that the chocolate cake would probably taste and smell good, and that it would be relaxing to take a break and eat it. However, when I look at what's behind the scene, what do I see? Where is eating this cake going to lead me? I see a number of possibilities, none of which are too appealing.

First of all, it's very likely that I'll feel sick or tired after eating the cake. Even if I don't, a very likely scenario is that it will lead me to the next piece of sugary food, and then to another, and on and on. This chocolate cake will probably stir up some strong sugar cravings for me in the future and will lead me right back down that road of addiction—a very painful path that I've been down before and don't want to travel again.

Once you become aware that there may be other scenarios behind the one you're seeing, it's a lot easier to pierce the illusion of the short-lived pleasure and find the other pictures that support your ultimate goals.

It can be tricky, because I may hear a voice that tells me, for example, "Just eat this one little piece . . . it can't possibly hurt you. This will be your last one. After you eat it, you absolutely won't have any more." It's time to recognize that these statements cause you to sabotage yourself. Every addict knows that thought: *This will be the last time I gamble* or *I'll only have one drink or one cigarette.*

Another common voice that often creeps in is the one that tells you: "You have no willpower. You'll never succeed." Often it's so familiar that you don't even challenge it. You lamely nod in agreement, silently reaffirming: *It's true, I have no willpower. I might as well give up any hope of ever being thin and in control of my life and my eating habits.* This thought then drives you to reach for that cake as if on automatic pilot.

I'm sure that you've heard these sabotaging voices one too many times. With the inner strength and fortitude that you'll be gathering as you continue to move through the Right Weigh program, you'll be able to easily turn to them and say, "No, I'm not listening to you." This is a lot easier to do when you're regularly tuning in to and listening to your own inner wisdom, the voice that does know and wants what's best for you.

This plan is about finding and following your own voice from deep in your core, and turning away from the old, harmful ones. You'll start to connect with the deeper reality within your heart, even if you're faced with an onslaught of negative statements. Remember: If you don't feed them with your attention, they'll disappear. Through the tools that you're being given, this can start to become second nature for you.

The first thing you need to do is become aware that the sabotaging voice is present and realize that it is, in fact, just a voice and nothing more. This puts some distance between you and it, which will naturally lessen its impact on you. Then you can tune in to how you're actually feeling in the moment.

When I return my focus to my body and its physical sensations, I may realize that the cake was so tempting to me because I'm really hungry. Then I can go inside myself and discover what my body actually needs—that is, what would support me right now? The choice doesn't have to be between miserable diet food that tastes like cardboard and some rich, tasty dish that's poisonous to my system. Instead, I can find healthful options that I really enjoy.

If I discover that I'm truly hungry, a picture of a big, delicious salad may come to mind—one with a fabulous dressing, maybe a few roasted pecans for flavor, goat cheese sprinkled on top, and probably some protein such as chicken or salmon. If I can tolerate sweetness, I may even chop a few figs or throw in some golden raisins along with a little freshly ground sea salt. I then have a delicious meal that satisfies my physical hunger *and* my desire for something tasty. When I check in with my body to see how I'm going to feel after I eat this, I get a strong *yes* signal, so I'll proceed to put it together.

On the other hand, I may tune in physically and realize that I'm not hungry at all, yet I really want to sit and eat this cake. At that point, I can take a moment and go behind the craving to discover what's going on inside. Maybe I'm experiencing stress or loneliness; or I'm feeling angry, overwhelmed, anxious, or bored. How can I offer myself the deepest support right now? This may be a wonderful time to practice the incredibly transformational tools of self-hypnosis, Remembrance, or prayer.

Then again, I may find by digging deeper and looking behind the picture of eating cake that what I really want is a warm bath, to get together with a good friend (not around food), or to step on the treadmill. Sometimes you may have such a narrow focus that you forget how many choices you have.

As you keep working with the Right Weigh program and develop the habit of looking inward and becoming more aware of the voices, pictures, and beliefs that are causing you to sabotage yourself and your desire to be thin, you'll learn to bring these to the light of your Creator so that they can be healed. Yes, it takes courage to examine yourself, but this is what will lead you to true freedom. By peeling away the layers of these false thoughts, you can start to get in touch with your true nature, your spirit of love and innocence.

Exercise 15: Silencing the Voices That Hold You Back

Think of a belief that keeps you stuck in the past or refer to one that you wrote down earlier. In your permanent-weight-loss journal, begin to write down all the voices you hear regarding this belief. Don't edit them—just write down what they say as they come into your awareness. Here are some that you might be hearing:

- "I'll never be thin."
- "I have no control."
- "I love chocolate."
- "I don't want to attract too much attention."
- "I need my weight for protection."
- "I won't give up ice cream."
- "This is too much work."
- "I just want to live my life the way I have been. It's not too bad."

Record This Exercise

Close your eyes. Take a deep breath in through your nose, hold it a moment, and exhale through your mouth, releasing any tension with the breath. Make sure that you're very grounded. Use your "cord" and sink those roots way down into the earth. Take the time to feel your hips, buttocks, and legs. You're traveling deep within your own being through the doorway of your heart.

Put your hand on your chest and take some long, slow, deep breaths, feeling the rise and fall. Imagine that emanating from the depths of your soul is the brightest, most radiant light you can envision. This symbolizes the highest intensity of love and wisdom in the Universe. Allow every pore of your skin and every fiber of your being to be bathed in this radiance. Imagine that your name for your Creator is written within this light.

Feeling the glow that springs forth from deep inside, slowly open your eyes and look at your list of voices. See the one that jumps out at you and has the most emotional impact. When you've picked it out, close your eyes again. Hear that voice and notice whether there's a picture associated with it. . . .

Take that statement and any image you associate with it and put them in your left hand. Just hold them there. Now, staying focused in your heart, place the name of your Creator, submerged in radiant light, in your right hand. If you haven't found a comfortable name, simply say "Aaaah" when you do this.

Really imagine the bright beams emanating from that higher vibration of the name in your right hand. If you don't see it, just feel it and get a sense of its awesome energy. When you're strongly connected to the greatest expression of power and love in the Universe, put your two hands together. Wash the voice and picture in your left hand with the greatness and strength of the light of the name of your Creator in your right hand. Continue to bring the name with the light around it to the voice until it is completely cleansed.

When you're ready, open your eyes and come back into the room.

Doing this exercise regularly will help you get into the positive habit of making space for all of the feelings that pop into your awareness. Trying to shut out the unwanted sensations or voices just makes those parts of yourself clamor for even more attention. Because you've shut out these parts of yourself, you've maintained the need to escape your feelings with food. Instead, allow your experience to be exactly what it is in the moment. By accepting all of your emotions, even the ones you may label "bad," you give them space to transform. Be present and give yourself gentleness and love.

Don't try to get rid of your thoughts—it's impossible. (Try not to think of a pink elephant and what comes to mind?) Rather than attempting to stop these thoughts, simply bring them to your inner Source and let this higher place show you what's true. If you give these harmful voices your attention by acknowledging them, however, you collude with them. So when you hear them, be firm and say, "No, I'm not listening to you. I've spent too much of my life being sucked in by you—now I'm choosing the voice of love and faith."

Exercise 16: Healing Through the Voices

In this exercise, you'll begin to wash the voices and pictures that don't serve you one by one, and in this way clean your heart. As you polish your core, it becomes a purer reflection of the truth of who you are, and less a projection of everything you've accumulated over your lifetime. (You don't need to record this exercise. Simply read it through once or twice and follow the instructions.)

Once again, go through the list of voices you wrote down in Exercise 15. Take them one at a time and ask your inner wisdom, the Source of Light, if there's anything you need to learn from the particular one you're working with. Don't be afraid to ask. Remember, it's only by doing so that you'll receive an answer. If you feel that you get no response, don't demand one; simply be patient and sit with it longer. Return to the quality of wisdom or the name of God written in light in your center and notice what comes into your awareness.

As insights come into your mind, write them down in your permanent-weight-loss journal in a different-color ink from the voices so that it's easy to differentiate them. For example, if your voice says, "I'm pathetic. I can't let anyone see how weak I am," write that down in blue. Bring this idea to the name of your Source and see what happens. Then, when you feel or hear a response, write down whatever you're shown in red or black, symbolizing your deeper guidance. Continue to do this with whatever voices come up for you at this time.

The more you can do this exercise with the attitude of a curious scientist, the greater benefit you'll derive from it. From a place of truly not knowing, ask your inner wisdom to show you the truth about this statement, even if you believe without a doubt that it's valid. Even if this is a voice that the people closest to you in the world would attest to, still bring it to the name of God in light. You're going inward, not looking for a consensus of opinion from those who know you. Remember, your outer world and the people in it often reflect your inner voices, no matter how unfounded they are, until you change those perceptions.

As you bring that idea to the name of God, perhaps you'll be shown a vision of your own beauty, the wonderful parent or friend that you are, some of the ways that you do exhibit strength and moderation, and all that you contribute.

By practicing bringing your beliefs to your higher wisdom and remembering your personal connection to the One, the Source of Life, the Divine Love, you'll begin to get a real sense that what seemed so real isn't solid at all. It's an illusion that you've been caught by and are therefore acting out. Some may have been passed down from generation to generation, or given to you by the culture, race, or religion you happened to be born into.

The Possibility of Healing Through the Exercises

When you're working with your emotions, internal images, and voices, as in the preceding exercises, it's important to realize that although sometimes the emotion just lifts and you're left with profound peace (or whatever quality you're working with), at other times there's a healing process, just as when you have a physical injury. So instead of living your life as a small person, step into the greatness of the Divine Source that wants to work through you.

Your Creator doesn't want you to suffer. You've been given the tools that you need to gain freedom—all you have to do is have the faith to use them and the perseverance to stick with this plan no matter what bumps you encounter along the road.

●●●●●

CHAPTER NINE

Step 5: Reprogram Your Subconscious Mind and Create Your Future

By now, you're very clear about what you don't want to be: overweight, out of control, addicted to food, or leading a sedentary lifestyle. You've visualized your outcome, turned to your Source for help, begun to accept yourself as you are, and started to break through the obstacles that have been holding you back. All of these steps involve a process, so even if you've only just begun to make progress with them, I hope that you'll stop and congratulate yourself for how far you've come and the positive momentum you've established so far.

It's now time to create the life you *do* want. Take out the vision that you wrote down in Step 1, look at the outcome you want, and let it really sink in. This is what you're beginning to create. You're transforming yourself into a person with positive eating habits—someone who's healthy, strong, fit, and at just the right weight.

The exercises in this chapter are based in self-hypnosis and neuro-linguistic programming (NLP). They'll help you discover and program into your brain the exact steps necessary to create what you desire. Albert Einstein is said to have remarked that a problem is never solved at the level it was created. What this means is that while you may spend a lot of time with your intellect, trying to solve life's challenges, you might realize at some point that you're simply repeating the same anxiety-provoking thoughts over and over . . . but not really coming up with anything useful. At those times it can be very helpful to put all that analysis aside, rest, and go to a deeper place in your being, beyond thought—another "level"—which is a place of unlimited creativity.

You may have heard that you only use 10 percent of your brain's capacity in daily life. Well, beyond your conscious mind lies the immense power of the subconscious, where habits and memories are stored, as well as the automatic functions of your body. In other words, if your mind were a huge iceberg, the conscious part would only be the tip. In order to create real and lasting change, you'll have to travel deeper and access the larger part of that iceberg: the subconscious.

Your old, unproductive habits of bingeing, snacking, having meals when you're not hungry, and emotional eating are deeply ingrained in this hidden portion of your consciousness, and as you work with this program, you'll actually be able to reprogram them. You won't need willpower because you won't be consciously overriding your thoughts.

When you use self-control, you force yourself to do something. But when the two parts of your mind are in harmony, you'll find yourself naturally doing things that lead to your heart's desire. For example, you know that you want to lose weight. And when your subconscious looks forward to daily physical activity and prioritizes it, both portions of your mind will work together to bring you closer to your goal.

The Subconscious and Habits

Your conscious mind knows that you can't keep on going the way you have been, and it really wants to change your life for the better. It has a burning desire for slenderness and health, and an equally strong fear of illness and disease. However, your unproductive habits regarding eating serve as a stimulus-response mechanism: It's as if a bell goes off in your environment, the thought of food comes in, and you respond automatically with unhealthy behaviors.

The subconscious part of you is like a computer, responding to the countless "bells" that are always sounding. It doesn't use logic or reasoning, simply running on "programs" and functioning automatically. It doesn't evaluate whether this makes sense or is good or bad.

It's like a garden—and you're the gardener. It's up to you to sow the kind of seeds that you want to flourish and grow. What thoughts do you want to plant? How do you want to direct your subconscious?

Even though there are an infinite number of choices you could make about what to think and do in any given moment, it's as if a pathway has been set up in your nervous system that makes you tend to repeat the same selections. The longer the pattern continues, the stronger the route in your nervous system becomes, much as a track in the snow gets tamped down the more people walk on it. This is why habits can be so difficult to break.

You know that you need to start eating smaller portions of healthier foods and increase your activity level, but it may seem as if you'll never get over your feelings of deprivation. And you may feel powerless when it comes to breaking painful associations with exercise. It isn't that you haven't put forth the effort, it's just that the task seems so overwhelming. You can stick to a diet for a period of time, but it may feel impossible to give up snacking and raiding the fridge at night forever.

The good news is that even the most deeply ingrained habits can be broken. Self-hypnosis and neuro-linguistic programming (NLP) are powerful tools you can use to plant new seeds in your mind that will lead to the results you desire.

Self-Hypnosis to Transform Old Habits

Hypnosis is a perfectly natural state, despite how it's often portrayed in the media. You actually go in and out of a light version of it throughout the day without even being aware of it. Have you ever driven someplace, and when you arrived, it felt as if only five minutes had passed . . . even though you might have been on the road for an hour? Yes, you were physically driving the car, but your mind drifted off somewhere else—into a mild hypnotic state. Another example is when you become so absorbed in reading a book or watching a movie that you don't hear the phone ringing or someone talking to you.

Hypnosis is simply a state of deep physical relaxation and focused concentration, in which the subconscious is more susceptible to suggestion. In fact, because we become so open in this condition, it's been used successfully as a substitute for anesthesia in dentistry, surgery, and even childbirth. Athletes use it all the time to get the "competitive edge"; and advertisers, who greatly understand the power of hypnotic suggestion, spend billions of dollars a year applying these principles to get consumers to buy their products. Now you can start to use this knowledge for your own benefit.

It can be surprising to realize how susceptible you really are. Try this fun exercise and see for yourself: Imagine walking into your kitchen, opening the refrigerator, and taking out a big, juicy lemon. Next, see yourself opening a drawer and taking out a knife. Slice the lemon, pick up a big piece, and suck on it—taste the sour juices.

Now come back to the present moment and notice your mouth—were you actually puckering, anticipating that sharp citrus taste? If you take the time to really visualize this scenario and not just think about it as an abstract concept, you'll automatically salivate because your subconscious doesn't know the difference between reality and imagination. When you envision new experiences, your mind will respond as if they're actually happening.

The Unexpected Benefits of Hypnosis

There are many remarkable physical and psychological benefits to hypnosis. The deeply relaxed state it induces (which is similar to meditation except that it's more goal-oriented) can relieve suffering from angina and arrhythmia. It may also lower blood pressure and cholesterol levels, enhance blood flow to the heart, and bolster the immune system. Research shows increased defenses against tumors, asthma, viruses, colds, flu, and other infectious diseases in people who regularly practice deep relaxation methods such as self-hypnosis. These techniques also block the negative effects of the stress hormone norepinephrine, which causes a racing heart, high blood pressure, anger, anxiety, and a greater vulnerability to pain. Regular practice often reduces backaches, migraines, and tension headaches, and may allow chronic-pain patients to reduce their reliance on painkillers.

There are also a wide range of psychological benefits, such as a decrease in neuroses and drug and alcohol abuse; and improved concentration, memory, and creativity. So just imagine the good things *you'll* experience if you begin regularly practicing self-hypnosis!

Of course, when it comes to achieving permanent weight loss, it's important to get into a deeply relaxed state so that you can receive the suggestions that will help you alter the way that you think about food. And when your thoughts change, so will your behavior. Think of it as downloading a new "program" onto your "hard drive"—an upgrade containing everything that you want to implement in your life.

As you practice the self-hypnosis in the next exercise, don't be concerned if it feels totally phony. You may tell yourself, "Small portions satisfy me," but hear a voice answering, "That's a lie!" Don't listen to it—you're going to challenge those destructive words directly.

Compounding Benefits with NLP

You're also going to learn neuro-linguistic-programming techniques to help you become aware of, and ultimately change, your internal pictures. NLP is a science that helps you access your nervous system—the mental pathways of your five senses—and work with language to reprogram the subconscious. It's very powerful because it helps you modify the way a scenario is stored in your memory, rather than focusing on its content. As the way things are stored in your brain changes, you'll notice a shift in your perception of the event. For example, you may remember a happy event in full color with sound and a warm feeling, whereas something sad might be stored in black and white or with fuzzy, dim images. Using NLP and self-hypnosis together can dramatically lessen the emotional impact of certain limiting beliefs and memories that may have kept you frozen in the past, diminishing your current choices when it comes to eating.

When your perspective shifts, your behaviors really will change. For instance, right now you may find it almost impossible to leave food on your plate. Deeply ingrained in your subconscious is the belief that you mustn't waste anything, which causes you to stuff yourself until you're uncomfortable. This is automatic for you, but when you practice self-hypnosis, your point of view will begin to shift. Childhood memories of being encouraged to clean your plate will lose their grip on you. You'll remember to stay in touch with your belly and notice when it's getting full—before your stomach is completely distended. You'll be able to walk away once you're no longer physically hungry, and it will be easy to ask for a take-out container to wrap up the rest of your meal when you're at a restaurant.

Or perhaps you have a program running that compels you to pull into fast-food places on a regular basis. When you practice self-hypnosis, you might discover that you associate a burger and fries with youth and freedom. Once you break those connections, you'll find yourself breezing past the drive-through without stopping.

By filling your brain with statements such as "I am no longer allowing myself to be the victim of each tempting, fattening food that comes along," while you're in a relaxed hypnotic state, you'll start to believe them and act as if they're true. The unconscious pictures that you've been holding for many years—seeing yourself as out of control, destined to be overweight, in a state of struggle, and always on a diet—will begin to be replaced by images of yourself as thin, healthy, energetic, preferring smaller portions, and fitting into your clothes comfortably.

Exercise 17: Self-Hypnosis to Create Your Future

Although self-hypnosis, much like meditation, is a wonderful way to relax the body and mind, in this book you're going to be using it specifically to reprogram your subconscious with suggestions to help you do what you consciously desire.

Before you record this exercise, make a list of the behaviors you'd like to eliminate, such as eating fast-food burgers and fries or drinking soda. Next, begin to create the positive self-talk that will have the greatest impact on you. Do this by writing down the new habits that you wish to incorporate into your lifestyle, such as carrying around healthy snacks, cooking rice and vegetables at home, and drinking water. Use the information you received from Exercise 13 to generate ideas.

After you've made both lists, write down the suggestions that you want to give yourself. These are positive affirmations, and as I mentioned, they work best when they're positive and in the present tense. Read through the list below and find the ones that resonate with you. It's also a good idea to create statements that are specific to your goals—and make sure to write them down. Some of your affirmations might be:

- *Small portions satisfy me.*

- *I enjoy working out at the fitness center. I particularly love the yoga classes.*

- *I reach for water throughout the day. I love its cool, clean taste. I look forward to all the benefits of drinking it.*

- *At parties, I concentrate on the people I get to socialize with.*

- *It is okay to throw away or wrap up the food my granddaughter leaves on her plate.*

- *I remember to carry healthy snacks with me. Celery is one of my favorites.*

- *I walk everywhere I can. I love the feeling of moving my body.*

- *I see myself thin and happy.*

- *I am absolutely determined to succeed.*

- *I am free from addiction. I only desire nutritious, wholesome foods.*

- *I love, respect, and care for my body.*

- *It feels so good when my stomach is slightly empty.*

- *I fit into my clothes comfortably.*

- *I love looking good.*

- *It is totally safe for me to look and feel good.*

- *I absolutely deserve to be healthy, fit, and attractive.*

- *I am in touch with my body and the foods it needs to feel good.*

- *I love to eat vegetables.*

- *It feels so good to be in control of my life and my eating habits.*

- *When I am tired, I can simply rest. I regulate my energy levels without food.*

- *I see myself at my ideal weight when I look in the mirror.*

- *I go through the day choosing healthy, nutritious foods.*

- *I reach for healthy snacks, such as fresh fruit between meals.*

- *I eat only when my body is physically hungry.*

- *I chew slowly, enjoying and appreciating every bite. I stop eating before my stomach is full.*

- *It is easy to incorporate physical activity into my daily life. I love walking* [or in-line skating or whatever activity I want to do].

- *I easily leave food on my plate.*

- *I am able to deal with my emotions directly, rather than submerging feelings with food.*

- *I am becoming healthier every day.*

- *I feel so much more comfortable as the weight comes off.*

- *I shed pounds easily and effortlessly.*

- *I am absolutely determined to live my life at my ideal weight.*

- *I am finished eating after dinner.*

- *I incorporate activity into all parts of my life.*

- *I am always prepared. I easily remember to have supplies on hand to prevent hunger.*

- *I avoid comparing myself with others. I love and care for myself.*

You'll begin with an induction, which is the technique used to get into the hypnotic state. Since this entire exercise is building the belief that you respond easily to suggestions, it's good to use an induction that works quickly. This will make you more accepting of the positive suggestions you'll be receiving.

While there are a variety of methods to choose from, one of my favorites is the eye-closure technique. You'll take a deep breath, close your eyes, and focus on the muscles around and behind them; then you'll instruct yourself to use your imagination and relax these muscles to the point where they *won't* work. It's very important to use the specific and explicit language provided below when giving yourself suggestions, because the subconscious takes things literally. When you're completely convinced that your eye muscles are *locked shut,* you'll give them a test to make sure that they won't function.

If your eyes pop open when you give them a try, that's okay. Remind yourself that the feeling of paralysis will be temporary—and only because *you* want it to happen. Simply begin again, this time just testing when you're really convinced that you can't move your eyes. After this, you'll feel the affected area relax, and you'll let that wave of calm flow through your whole body, all the way down to your toes.

This induction is a wonderful way to convince your conscious mind that it's responding to suggestion. Once you believe that you're in a state of hypnosis, your subconscious will more readily accept what it's being told. You'll have succeeded in bypassing the conscious mind's ability to assess information critically and decide whether to reject it.

During this process, your logic won't disappear; it's always with you. If there were an emergency, you'd immediately "come to" so that you could attend to the situation. However, this frame of mind is so pleasant that most people prefer to stay there as long as possible. And it's important for you to remember that you're always in complete control and can emerge at any time. When you want to come back, it's a good idea to count slowly from one to five so that you have plenty of time to integrate the experience into your normal consciousness.

Remember, hypnosis isn't sleep; it's a state of relaxed alertness. You'll be aware of your surroundings and even have a sense of heightened awareness. It's natural for thoughts to come into your mind; if they do, simply bring yourself back to the sound of your voice on the recording or to the suggestions that you're hearing. If you find yourself falling asleep, practice sitting up instead of lying down.

You can memorize the following self-hypnosis induction, but it will probably be easier if you read it into a tape recorder and then play it back. After you've recorded it, you'll continue the guided imagery by reading through the affirmations you've selected from the list or personally created. If you've gained insight about specific new behaviors that you'd like to adopt from the earlier exercise when you contacted your inner wisdom, be sure to incorporate those into this script.

Finally, you'll give yourself the post-hypnotic direction to embed the suggestions you give yourself more firmly into your mind. In this case, you'll be saying that every time you see the color green, you become more and more responsive to your affirmations and positive images, and your commitment to your goals will be strengthened. This can have a dramatic effect on your success, since green is everywhere—traffic lights, vegetables, trees, and plants—and will act as a constant reminder of the personal outcome you're moving toward. Also, green means go—moving forward—and that's exactly what you're doing.

This exercise will take approximately 20 minutes, but you can shorten it by skipping the part where you deepen the hypnosis by imagining a star. When you do the section with the imagery of food and living at your ideal weight, you might want to tailor it with specific pictures that will resonate for you.

Record This Exercise

Get as comfortable as possible, then find a point on the ceiling to look at, take a deep breath . . . hold it a moment . . . exhale and close your eyes. Relax your body as much as possible as you take another deep breath and hold it . . . and slowly exhale, allowing any remaining tension to leave your body with the air.

Bring your awareness to all of the muscles behind and around your eyes. Relax your eyes and the surrounding areas to the point that they won't work. Use your imagination and pretend that your eye muscles are so relaxed that they just *won't work*. Pretend that no matter how hard you try, they just won't function. When you're absolutely *convinced* that your eyes are completely *locked shut*, go ahead and test them. . . . Give them a good try . . . and stop testing.

Just let your eye muscles relax. Allow that wave of relaxation to flow from them into your entire head. . . . Imagine a radiant, colored light dropping in through the top of your skull and filling it, relaxing every muscle, fiber, and cell. Visualize this brilliant glow traveling down your neck and throat, bringing soothing relaxation, then continuing into your shoulders, arms, hands, and fingers, all the way down to your fingertips.

See the color filling your entire torso and upper, middle, and lower back, permeating every muscle, organ, and bone . . . absorbing any tension. This beautiful hue is flowing down into the chair or bed supporting you. Feel your body sink, and allow yourself to be held as you relax all of the muscles in your pelvis. The light continues down through your legs . . . into your thighs, knees, calves, ankles, feet, and toes. Imagine any remaining stress leaving your body through the soles of your feet. Envision the earth absorbing it, and just let it sustain you.

To become more grounded, imagine a cord of light from your belly button reaching all the way down into the center of the earth; it can be any thickness you desire. Imagine it taking root in the center of the earth, connecting you to your home.

In a moment, you'll be able to open and close your eyes. And when they shut again, allow your relaxation to double. You don't need to try to figure this out—just allow your subconscious to do it for you, and accept its gift. This will happen for only one reason: because you want it to. So in a moment you can count to three and open your eyes. . . .

One . . . two . . . three . . . open your eyes . . . and close them. Let your body become twice as relaxed. Feel all your muscles go loose and limp like a rag doll.

In a moment you can once again count to three and open your eyes . . . and close. And when your eyelids drop, allow yourself to unwind even further and become twice as relaxed as you are right now. This will happen because you want it to. So on the count of three, open your eyes . . . one . . . two . . . three . . . and close your eyes . . . feel your relaxation doubling . . . and enjoy the peaceful feelings. . . .

Now that your body is deeply relaxed, you can also relax your mind. There's nothing you need to do right now. If thoughts come into your head, simply allow them to pass, like clouds in the sky of your vast mind . . . and return to your breathing . . . revel in the sensations. Enjoy the pleasure of keeping your eyes closed.

In a few moments, you'll begin to count down from ten to one, becoming more and more peaceful as you go, dropping down even deeper into the calm. As you say each number, you'll see it in your mind's eye, perhaps written in the sand at the beach or on a chalkboard. So listen as I speak and count with me, going deeper and deeper into a hypnotic state with each number. Ten . . . relaxing more and more . . . nine . . . going deeper and deeper . . . eight . . . calming further. . . seven . . . going down . . . six . . . all feelings are very peaceful . . . five, four, three . . . almost there now . . . two . . . and one . . . very deeply relaxed. . . .

I want you to imagine that you're looking up into a beautiful night sky and that you can see a star in the distance. You spy one beautiful silver light, shining down out of a velvety black sky, and it's millions of miles away. Focus your gaze entirely on that solitary star. . . . And as you do so, you notice it beginning to twinkle, and you become more and more relaxed . . . more peaceful . . . more calm.

As you gaze at the star, you feel yourself becoming sleepier and drifting deeper. From time to time, you may almost feel like you're dropping off to sleep because you're so relaxed . . . so relaxed . . . so relaxed. . . .

Imagine yourself as you truly desire to be. You're standing in front of a mirror and seeing your reflection gazing back at you, at your ideal weight. You're looking and feeling your absolute best. You feel a greater level of self-confidence than ever before.

See yourself naturally choosing nutritious, water-rich, unprocessed foods. Fresh Boston lettuce bursting with vitamins . . . crisp orange carrots crunching as you bite down . . . bright red cherry tomatoes, filled with juice . . . perfectly grilled salmon flaking as you pierce it with a fork. . . . Smell the nutty aroma of flaxseed oil as you drizzle it on a salad . . . and feel the satisfaction in your mouth as you taste salads, vegetables, lean protein, and whole grains. . . . Use all of your senses in this visualization. Make sure that you see the colors around you—vivid, bright, close, and clear.

You're succeeding. You're in control of your life and eating habits, and are achieving your ideal weight!

And now you see a huge, gloppy serving of scalloped potatoes in front of you. The greasy butter is dripping from it, and the grayish-yellow color is disgusting to you. You're pushing the plate away, exhaling the repulsive odor from your nose as you shove it far from you. Visualize your blood flowing through your arteries freely now that you've rejected that food.

Imagine that you're feeling better than ever now, and looking forward to being active each and every day. See and feel yourself engaging in a sport or activity that you really enjoy. You feel terrific as you move your body. You're sweating—and it feels great! As you exercise, you're breathing deeply. It feels so good to be alive! Upsets and irritations bounce off you as you relish your new relationship with your body and your life. . . .

From now on, every time you see the color green, you'll experience yourself totally in control of your life and your eating habits, feeling wonderfully relaxed and happy. This will happen without effort on your part. When you see green trees, lawns, signs, traffic lights, fabric, vegetables—anything green at all—you'll smile as you have a visceral experience of being relaxed and in control . . . selecting healthy meals naturally, leaving food on your plate, and choosing to enjoy some exercise on a regular basis.

The color green reminds you to see and feel this state of confidence regarding the positive changes occurring in your life. Green brings to mind your new commitment to your health. When you see any hue from lime to emerald, you'll remember to take a moment and find the place in your heart that's absolutely committed to achieving slenderness and living a happier, healthier life. . . .

I'm going to count from one to five, and bring you up out of this state of peace. All feelings of drowsiness will completely disappear, and you will return wide awake and wonderfully refreshed. One . . . you're beginning to come up . . . two . . . feeling refreshed and alert. . . three . . . retaining all of your blissful feelings . . . four . . . embracing every new teaching . . . and five—wide awake!

It's a good idea to let yourself emerge slowly so you can fully integrate the benefits. Each time you do this exercise, allow yourself to go even deeper into the hypnotic state.

The more you practice self-hypnosis techniques and modify your inner dialogue, the more ingrained these changes will become. Over time, the concepts and language from the suggestions and images will become a part of who you are.

Exercise 18: Changing Your Perceptions of Pleasure and Pain

Here's a quick little exercise that will help you break the association of pleasure with a food that you really want to stop eating (there's no need to record this).

Close your eyes and imagine a food that you absolutely love to eat, but that you want to stop having because you know it's harmful. Mentally place this in your left hand.

Now look at it and see it in black and white, appearing fuzzy and drab. Take as much time as you need to get this image or sense of the unwanted item.

Visualize a food that you strongly dislike in your right hand—make sure that it's something you despise (or at least feel very negatively toward). See it as best you can in full, bright color, then bring it in very close. Smell it fully and imagine tasting the disgusting flavor.

When you're ready, put your hands together. Watch the two foods— the one that you crave in black and white on the left, and one that you can't stand in full color on the right. With your hands joined, see all the flavors and smells blending to make one food. Imagine eating it—what does it taste like?

Spend a few minutes with your eyes closed, really imagining that item that you used to desire, covered with the juices or flavors of the one you loathe . . . see them completely blended.

When done properly, this exercise is very powerful. Many of my clients find that they only need to do it once in order to achieve a strong, negative reaction to the food they used to crave. However, it's something that you can be practiced as often as necessary to produce the desired result.

Exercise 19: Changing Your Internal Pictures

In this exercise, you'll look at the hidden pictures you hold inside that sabotage your quest to achieve your goals and create the future you desire. You'll start by writing in your permanent-weight-loss journal and then move on to the guided meditation (which you'll record).

Take a moment and write down the assumptions that you know are blocking your success. To do this, think of the obstacles that get in your way of achieving and maintaining your ideal weight—for instance, perhaps you're around food all the time because of the kind of work you do. Answering these questions will help you discover more scenarios that may be slowing your progress.

- Do the people around you encourage you to have certain dishes that you know aren't the best choices?

- Do you find yourself eating alone late at night, after everyone else has gone to bed?

- Do you associate food with relaxation, privacy, comfort, and pleasure?

- Do you consume most of your calories socially—such as at parties or when you go out to dinner?

- Do you eat as a way to keep yourself awake or energized?

- Do you snack when you're upset, as a way to change your emotions?

Take a moment to write down your greatest obstacles or use one that you noted in Exercise 13. For example, you may discover a belief that if you don't eat something right away, it will be all gone later; or that it's not safe to be thin because you'll attract too much sexual attention. You might become aware that you think it's wrong to throw food away. Perhaps you have the feeling that you don't deserve to be in shape. Write down anything you become conscious of that's caused you to eat.

Record This Exercise

Close your eyes, take a few deep breaths, and allow yourself to sink down into the chair or bed. Do a quick mental scan of your body, notice any part that feels tight or constricted, and breathe gently into that area. Spend an extra moment scanning your pelvic region, belly, shoulders, upper back, and jaw—all places where you may hold tension. If you feel any constriction, send that part of yourself some love and relaxation.

Open your eyes briefly and choose one of the obstacles that you wrote down to work with. Close your eyes and imagine the scenario to the best of your ability. See what picture comes to your mind when you think of that situation. If there's no visual, just notice any feelings, sensations, or voices.

Look at the image you have of yourself, the one that's been blocking your success. As you look at the picture, notice the hues. . . . If it's in color, change it to black and white. . . . If it's panoramic, stretching on and on, put a frame around it. . . . Change it from focused to fuzzy and make a three-dimensional picture flat. Put some distance between you and that place. See it shrinking . . . and notice how doing this reduces some of its power.

If there's a texture to the picture, change it: Play with making it rough, smooth, soft, or even bumpy. If you're aware of a temperature—hot or cold—switch it. If you hear anything, turn down the volume to make the sounds very soft. . . . Change the characters' voices to a "Mickey Mouse" tone, or something equally ridiculous.

If you're experiencing the scenario through your own eyes, experiment with seeing yourself *in* the action, as if you're viewing a photo of yourself. . . . Now put a frame around it, and notice what happens when you make these changes. Does the memory seem different somehow? Take time to observe any internal shifts in your response to the obstacle you're working with.

When you're ready, open your eyes and come back into the room.

Many people notice that even the most upsetting events take on less importance when they change the way the memories are stored by exaggerating or diminishing the actual image, feeling, and sound.

When you alter the nuances of your internal representations, their impact changes. For instance, if you recall an unpleasant incident in full color, this may increase the emotional charge. However, when it goes to black and white, you may feel more in control. When you recall your child screaming, you may notice that your body tightens up and you want to go straight for the ice cream, but when you put the tune of "Yankee Doodle" in the background, you won't react so strongly to that outburst. This is a component of NLP known as *sub-modality changing.*

Using this technique can have a dramatic effect on the negative memories that you may be holding on to. By altering the way you remember something—whether it's near or far, bright or dim, or with or without sound—you can soften or eliminate the detrimental impact old pictures may be having. If you find this helpful, practice using it with other items on your list.

Exercise 20: Mental-Movie Reprogramming

In this exercise, you'll imagine seeing yourself in a movie theater, watching the painful event or unwanted behavior on the big screen. By distancing yourself from the "film," you're dissociating from it, therefore reducing its emotional impact. You can watch and learn what you need to, without having to relive the unpleasant drama.

For example, let's say I become aware that I love to eat at night after everyone else goes to bed. To start the exercise, I'd make a mental movie of myself bingeing on potato chips and sour cream at night. Rather than associating with the picture, I'd put it up on a movie screen. Then I'd imagine that I'm up in the projection booth, looking down at myself in the audience, who's watching the film of me pigging out. I'd let the entire movie run—from the anticipation of the pleasure of those chips, to unconsciously eating half the bag, to feeling sick and regretful as I crawl into bed.

At that point, it's helpful to watch the show again, only this time in slow motion and then again at high speed. If I want, I can do this three or four times, all the while remaining up in the projection booth, observing myself down in the audience, looking at the screen. As you discovered earlier, a lot can be learned from a situation by witnessing it without the associated feelings.

This process helps make your unproductive habits conscious and lessens the emotional impact of past traumatic events. In a moment, you'll do this exercise using one of your unwanted eating behaviors as the content of the movie.

Don't concern yourself with doing this "right." Even if you have difficulty seeing the images on-screen or imagining yourself in the projection booth *and* looking at yourself watching the movie, pretend that you're able to do it. Just setting your intention can be powerful, even if you aren't consciously aware of any visual component.

You'll find that the more you view yourself performing an unhelpful action in a disassociated or bizarre way (slow motion, high speed, watching yourself as a spectator), the more aware you'll be. This will collapse your conviction that "this just is how I am," because you'll gain perspective. The next time you start to harm yourself in that way, you'll be more aware of the triggers and more likely to respond differently. Your subconscious habits will shift.

If you have one particularly troublesome habit, you can repeat this exercise as much as you need to. You can determine how long to work with it based on your behavioral changes. For example, if I notice that I no longer want those chips at night, and instead find myself taking a long walk in the evening before bed, I know that I don't need to work with that sequence anymore.

Bring to mind a situation related to your overweight condition that upsets you. For example, you may believe that you need chocolate to feel good and for comfort. So every time you experience even the least amount of stress or discomfort, you find yourself reaching for the candy, only to feel remorseful afterward. When you write down "I need chocolate," wait and see what comes up.

Perhaps the next thought that moves into your awareness is a time that you had an unpleasant exchange with a loved one, so you reached for your favorite crutch. The mental movie in this case may be getting angry at your partner, then sneaking off to the kitchen and taking out the hidden bag of miniature candy bars. You open them and stick them in your mouth, just as you hear your mate coming downstairs calling your name—then you quickly hide the wrappers in the garbage so that he won't see them. This would be the scene you'd work with.

Record This Exercise

Close your eyes, take a couple of deep breaths, and settle in. Ground down into the earth with the imaginary cord extending down from your belly. Strengthen your connection by visualizing this cord to be as wide as a telephone pole. Feel your legs and imagine that you have deep roots connecting you with the earth.

See the scenario in front of you on a movie screen. Imagine that you're seated in the audience, about to watch the show. As it begins, float up to the projection booth and watch yourself sitting in the audience, viewing the feature. Witness yourself acting out the scene, whether it's a specific memory, habitual behavior, or inner conflict. . . . Run through the entire thing.

Now observe yourself looking at the same events in slow motion (you're still in the projection booth). . . . And as this show ends, start it again from the beginning, this time played at high speed. Your thoughts and the sounds you hear go by lightning fast. . . . Repeat this, all the while staying in the projection booth, watching yourself, watching the film: at high speed again . . . then normally . . . and finally in slow motion. . . .

Whenever you're ready, open your eyes.

Think of the event that was troublesome to you earlier. Does it feel different for you now? Perhaps as you did this exercise, you realized that even though the situation was very familiar and had left you with a bad feeling, you could begin to see the humor in it—or have more compassion for yourself. Maybe you became aware of a better way to handle it. For example, if your picture had been of yourself sneaking chocolate after a fight with your lover, you might realize that you should have spoken to him and communicated your feelings directly.

Now that you're learning new ways to handle stress, manage your moods and energy level, draw upon your inner resources, and find perspective as you become more aware of the Truth within, you'll be able to see how to change this habit. You now have some incredibly simple yet powerful methods for taking care of yourself and getting centered when you feel out of balance, slip into old behaviors, or are jarred by your environment and emotional reactions. From this place of internal connection, you'll move toward achieving the state of slenderness, fitness, and control that you long for.

CHAPTER TEN

Step 6: Letting Go of the Past

Many of the habits that you repeatedly engage in have been with you since childhood. When you were young, you might have been trained to clean your plate. If you did, you were most likely rewarded with more food, especially dessert. Was this the way that your parents showed love? Although their intent wasn't malicious—they only wanted you to grow up big and strong—the result is that you're literally programmed to finish all the food you're served.

Were you ever encouraged to listen to your body and its signals about hunger? Did your parents (or caregivers) teach you to stop eating before you were totally satiated, understanding that it sometimes takes the brain a little while to register that the stomach is full? Chances are that you didn't learn to trust yourself.

You were inadvertently taught to ignore your bodily sensations, eat everything on your plate, and even have seconds so that you could be labeled "good" by the people you relied on and cared about the most. Rather than thinking that you're a failure today because of your size, you can say that you're a very good learner. When you reframe it in that way, you'll realize that you have the potential to learn new, positive behaviors that support your deepest desires for yourself and your life.

Staying on Track

Sometimes you may veer off course, but now you know where you're heading and that it's possible to get right back on track. So if Part I and the steps you've done so far have helped you determine that you need to avoid sugar, it's still okay if you just had a cookie. You'll understand that it doesn't mean you have to eat the entire box. After all, if you were carrying a tray of glasses and one fell off and broke, you wouldn't say to yourself, *Oh well, I might as well drop the whole tray!* Whenever you stray from your new path, have the utmost compassion and mercy for yourself. Your number-one support person is you.

Naturally, you'll still want to enjoy eating. When you're maintaining your ideal weight, you'll actually be able to enjoy food even more, because you won't be obsessed with it. You'll use it as a way of maintaining your life, since what you take in is the fuel for your body.

You wouldn't dream of filling your home with trash. Why then would you routinely fill your body—the home for your spirit and personality—with garbage that lacks any nutritional value? Your physical being is a holy gift from God. It's okay to regret how you've treated yourself without feeling bad or wrong for doing so. If you were driving somewhere and realized that you'd made a wrong turn, you'd simply go back, acknowledging that you'd made a mistake.

By the same token, you've made errors in certain areas of your life. Perhaps the priorities you set weren't for your highest good; maybe you valued a certain taste or pleasing someone more than your health and well-being. Praying and asking for forgiveness from your loving Father/Mother God will allow you to correct your course and return to the original state of love and compassion—for both yourself and others—that you had at birth.

The wrong turns you've made may have originated 30 or 40 years ago when your mind was first programmed with thoughts such as: *Finish everything put in front of you* or *Have a piece of candy—you'll feel better.* As a child, you were obviously too young to know any better, and you weren't in a position to challenge these concepts. However, the mistake was repeating this unproductive programming for so many years, and now it's time to move on.

Forgiveness

You may have difficulty forgiving yourself. Perhaps you harbor ill feelings for the years you've spent consuming the wrong foods, bingeing, snacking, eating for emotional reasons, and being inactive. You may even feel resentment toward significant people in your life such as your parents, grandparents, siblings, or spouse, who you may feel have contributed to your current dilemma. Maybe you can even remember specific events or comments that propelled you into eating with wild abandon and giving up on yourself.

You have to heal these wounds in order to take control of your eating and exercising. You may be very successful in many other areas of your life, but if you still see yourself as weak, helpless around food, or needing to get even with certain people, then you're the captain of a sinking ship.

Maybe there's something that you feel you can never forgive yourself for. By holding on to this guilt, you'll stay stuck in helplessness and negativity. These memories literally suck your life force away, diminishing your energy and quality of life—and they can ultimately lead to illness.

How can you possibly absolve yourself or others? You may have been physically or emotionally abused or mistreated, past events might have left you deeply wounded and scarred, or perhaps you feel incredibly guilty for some of your own actions. Forgiveness doesn't imply that you condone any of that. It simply means that you finally get to let go of the impact past events are having on your life today. . . . It means freedom.

Even if you had loving parents and an ideal childhood, you may be holding on to painful memories that you aren't even aware of. When you recall how open and impressionable you were as a child, you may realize that it would be almost impossible to go through life thus far without having your heart hurt in one way or another. Unfortunately, when that happens, your tendency is to shut down and contract, thereby blocking the natural flow of compassion. It's at those times when you felt cut off from love that you may have learned to soothe yourself with food. When you examine these recollections and transform them by using the Right Weigh program, you'll be able to forgive and let go of the past.

Don't worry: You aren't being asked to do this all on your own. You're going to go deep inside your heart and reconnect with your Source, Who's an endless font of mercy.

TAPPING IN TO DIVINE FORGIVENESS

You may have heard that God is all-forgiving, and this is true. When you tap in to your Source, it's easier to clearly understand any lessons from the past and have a better perspective about your life. You may even discover that the most painful events are the ones that ultimately set you free.

If you feel that you're nowhere near ready to see the positive aspects of your experiences, that's okay. You may not always be given the insight into why things happen as they do, yet through the exercises presented here, you'll gain much more inner peace and begin to reclaim your life.

Turning to God doesn't mean that you can expect Him to just miraculously heal all your inner wounds and turn your life around with no effort on your part. The old adage is true: God helps those who help themselves. When you show your Creator your absolute commitment to change and humility and express a willingness to set aside any fears or skepticism, you can be sure that you'll get assistance. Your Source loves you more than you care for yourself and is as close as your next breath, so open up to this Truth within you.

No matter what you've been through in the past or what actions you've taken that cause you immense regret and guilt, know that God is with you now, and always has been. Where was the Source of Life when these events were happening? Holding you. If you look back, you'll most likely see the angels who were there for you: the people who showed up to help, even if it was nothing more than a stranger pushing your car out of the snow or giving you good directions to get back on the freeway. To truly forgive—especially if you aren't sure it's possible—you must tune in to the Divine.

It's quite natural to not want to let go of the past when you've been deeply hurt or abused, and you don't need to force yourself to do so. Instead, you can allow the quality of forgiveness from a Higher Source to permeate your being. Over time, the impact of the traumatic incidents will decrease, and it will be easier to let go of your emotional attachments to them.

RETURNING TO LOVE

You're not asking for forgiveness because you're bad or wrong, but simply because you wish to be returned to your natural state of love; it hurts to be cut off from it. Although you may be positive that your suffering has been induced by the event and its perpetrator, in reality the pain is sustained by your inability to let go and return to the harmony of your essential nature. Anytime you deviate from this, you'll be constricted; when you return to it, you'll feel expansion. This is the internal barometer for your consciousness. You certainly won't condone other people's abusive, rude, or inappropriate behavior. You'll simply break free from its crippling effect on your life. And when it seems impossible to find the Divine, you can turn within and pray for help.

When you're practicing the next exercise, you may sometimes feel the opposite of forgiving or loving. If you find yourself disconnected and in a place of anger and judgment, don't despair. Instead, practice the Remembrance exercise, sincerely call on the qualities you desire, and let the higher vibration from them cleanse your heart and soul. If your conscious mind has difficulty understanding what that means, don't be concerned. Simply being open to transformation will help you heal.

Your harsh emotions don't make you wrong or bad, just human, so resist the urge to push them aside. The more you try to shut them off, the longer you'll have them. It's okay if you're in a place of pain, even though it doesn't feel good. Just start exactly where you are.

The following exercise will help you break through to a place of greater insight and peace. Accept what you're actually experiencing in the moment, and be gentle with yourself. If you encounter a strong emotion, it's probably a reaction to one of your beliefs, so take the time to explore it. For example, ask yourself, *What am I angry about?* Give yourself the space to let your unpleasant state of mind move and be transformed.

Exercise 21: Forgiveness

You may find yourself shouting or crying, so you might want to choose a time and place to do this where you're certain you won't be disturbed. It's important that you don't hold in your response.

You'll be calling in the light of the Divine as a source of forgiveness. When you do so, address your Higher Power by saying "God, the Great Forgiver" or whatever makes you feel comfortable.

Record This Exercise

Get very comfortable, close your eyes, and take a couple of deep breaths, letting any tension from the day leave your body. Relax your jaw and allow your pelvic muscles to loosen up, as you let yourself just sink down into your chair.

Focus on your center and begin to repeat the name of God in your heart, whether it's one from a religious tradition or simply the sound "Aaaah." Next, bring to mind the person you're having difficulty forgiving (if it's you, see yourself there in front of you), then mentally pull that image into your heart.

Visualize the name of your Source written in light in the air in front of you, then move it inside you, placing it over the picture in your heart. Now imagine the word *forgiveness* etched in light and hovering before you. Bring it within and superimpose it on the forms that are already there.

If you find yourself getting upset, just experience your emotions, whatever they are. If you feel angry or hurt by this person, it's okay; if you want to scream, cry, or yell, go ahead. But as you do so, continue to call on the radiance of the Divine that resides within you. Stay focused and let the power of forgiveness ride on your breath and permeate your core.

Appeal to the highest light you can imagine as you're saying the name and summoning forgiveness. Merge your Source's name and the higher attribute with the picture of the person you're having trouble forgiving. Allow the brilliance to fill, and flow through, the picture you're working with, and stay with this process until you notice an internal shift.

When you're ready, come back into the room.

This exercise allows you to wash away painful relics of the past, although you may need to work with the same person or event several times before it clears completely.

Exercise 22: Growing from Mistakes

Make a list of all your current behaviors concerning food or activities that you feel have caused you to gain weight. Don't judge yourself, because there's no room for that in your new life—only for the sincere desire to change and start over again. You're going to ask for help in learning from your mistakes and wiping the slate clean so that you can have what you truly desire.

If you grow from your failures, you'll become strong; but if you pretend they didn't happen, try to justify them, or spend a lot of time feeling bad, they won't benefit you at all. Looking at your past opens you to the choices (and consequences) that are available now. You aren't horrible for saying, "I've cheated on my diet, so I might as well just continue and eat everything in the house." But your new statement might be: "Okay, I just ate two cookies. I wish I hadn't done that, but I did. Now I'm going to have a carrot and a glass of lemon water and go out for a walk. Then I'll spend 30 minutes in prayer and Remembrance, letting myself feel the Peace of the Higher Realms."

Follow these steps in order to fully examine each mistake and begin learning from it:

1. In your permanent-weight-loss journal, make a list of the behaviors regarding food that you regret.

2. Ask yourself for forgiveness from the deepest part of your being that you can access.

3. Look inside and see when your moments of vulnerability are likely to occur in the future. Choose healthy habits as substitutes.

4. Commit to not repeating these mistakes in the future, while accepting that perfection is impossible.

It can also be helpful to practice the above exercise while looking in the mirror. Truly radiate mercy and compassion to yourself.

The Power of Prayer to Transform You

Every thought is a prayer—particularly those that are fueled by strong emotions. When you think, *I'll never get over what happened to me, I'll never lose this weight,* or *I can't believe how fat I am—I look awful!* with disgust, you're implanting these ideas as reality in your subconscious. And although you may be overweight, it doesn't have to be your destiny.

No matter what happened in the past, the vast power of your Creator is inside you, and you can tap in to this incredible force for change. When you pray from your center, you'll begin to experience more profound levels of peace and happiness than you ever thought possible. You'll access the part of yourself that's connected to everything and everyone beyond the hurt of past events, and you'll know exactly what actions you need to take in order to permanently achieve your ideal weight.

This doesn't necessarily happen when you pray sporadically for a particular change. But when you adopt a consistent, specific prayer plan that's designed to help you let go of the past and move forward to your fullest potential, you'll begin to see shifts in your life.

This isn't a way of doing nothing and saying "You handle it, God," as you continue to behave in the same old, unproductive ways. Instead, it's making a commitment to yourself to do whatever's necessary to manifest the Higher Will for your life. This will link you to the Divine spark within so that you can find the clarity and strength to take action. You'll return to your original state of wholeness, love, beauty, and joy, allowing you to recognize your true worth.

Of course, there isn't just one way to pray, and you'll need to find a style that's comfortable for you. However, being unsure of how to go about it often becomes an excuse for not reaching out at all.

HOW THE DIVINE WORKS TO HELP US

Each of us is like a lamp, and God is the electricity. Through prayer, you'll plug yourself in to the flow of love, forgiveness, power, compassion, wisdom, and strength from your Creator. You'll discover that the Universe is a living, eternal presence that responds to you. Although this Force will always remain a mystery, your life will be uplifted by developing a strong, personal relationship with your Source.

It's true that there's no formula for getting what you want—God's will may be greater than what you're asking for. For example, you may want to keep from being tempted by chocolate, and the answer could be that you'll happen upon a health-food store with marvelous produce. As you learn to trust the Universe, you may start eating vegetables, and the more you do, the more you'll notice that your taste is changing. You'll find that you prefer the flavor of steamed zucchini and yellow squash to candy bars, and you'll get in touch with how much lighter you feel. So instead of being turned off by chocolate, you'll get turned on by vegetables.

When you're willing to give up control of the *how* and *when* of losing weight, you'll open up to the unlimited potential of the Universe and the many ways that good can manifest. You'll truly begin to trust the prayer: "Thy will, not mine, be done."

In the past, you may not have seen ways to exercise, get healthy food, or find time to cook; but when you get in touch with Spirit, all kinds of opportunities will appear. You'll decide that you've had enough abuse at your job and find a new one that's not only better, but which also gives you more free time, letting you get up and walk around during the day instead of always sitting at your desk. You'll release fast food, and voilà, a farmers' market will open up in your neighborhood, where you'll discover a delicious variety of vegetables and herbs—and vendors who are happy to tell you how to store and cook their products.

Perhaps you'll let go of someone who doesn't support you in your goals, and then meet someone who eagerly invites you to take up jogging so that the two of you can run together (instead of encouraging you to indulge in happy hour as a form of after-work rebellion). These are new things that will come when you let go of the old. Sometimes the connection is obvious, but sometimes it isn't. You'll just make the shift and the Universe will respond in a mysterious way.

OPENING UP TO HOPE

When you connect with God, miracles happen. Sometimes they're small and make you think, *How odd!* such as discovering the farmers' market just after praying for help losing weight. Sometimes they're huge, such as being able to tolerate a very painful confrontation at a family holiday party: You may respond by going within and praying, and end up *not* reaching for food as a way to calm and nurture yourself.

How can you know that miracles exist? Look at the wonder of life all around you. If the blessing of a birth can occur daily, people can be healed of chronic illness against all odds, your body can function with such precision, and a tiny seed can become a beautiful rose or a great redwood, how can the miracle of your ideal weight not be possible? Habits such as bingeing, snacking, and emotional eating can be transformed not just through changing your subconscious programming and making a sincere commitment, but also through prayer.

Exercise 23: Personal Affirmative Prayer

When you turn to God for help, you'll surrender your ego completely and listen to what your Creator says. Messages may come to you in the form of thoughts, pictures, songs, the words of strangers or friends, or movies . . . the possibilities are unlimited. Perhaps you've turned on the radio and heard the lyrics to a song that spoke directly to you. You may not even be aware of all the times that your prayers are answered spontaneously, so do your best to be completely open with God. Pray regularly, as described here and in Chapter 6, and pay attention to messages from your Source that may come in unexpected ways.

Here are seven insights into the process of affirmative prayer (which you'll be doing in this exercise):

1. Be honest about where you are. Share your tears, weaknesses, and vulnerabilities with your Higher Power. Don't try to be positive or act happy or strong. When you show your weakness and fear, God can come to those places within you that need love, compassion, and strength. It's through your deepest suffering that you can come to know and feel how loved you are, but only when you have the willingness to "give it to God." Show your pain, confide your troubles, and say with the utmost sincerity, "Please help me and show me how you see this. I feel weak and needy. What's Your perspective?" It's safe to reveal your tears and to pray from your heart.

2. Let God enter into your soul. Really receive the outpouring of Divine love that pours forth automatically when you appeal for help—even if you doubt if it's real. Breathe the healing into the place inside you that feels a sense of lack, limitation, or discomfort. Know that no matter how powerful the unpleasant emotion or physical sensation, this light is even stronger. The best way to access the sacred is through your heart, so imagine that you can actually inhale this higher love through that core.

3. Ask God for what you want. This doesn't mean that you should ask for what your outer ego may desire (for instance, to look better than someone else). Instead, you should request the true longings of your soul. Ask God to help you fulfill your purpose and receive all the blessings that are here for you. Seek the truth of who you are— your beauty, your love, and the sanctity of your body, which serves as a vessel for your soul here on Earth. Appeal for help honoring your body and knowing what steps you need to take to achieve health at every level.

Be honest about the likelihood that your overweight condition is a symptom of an unhealed belief or emotion. Your goal is to heal that obstacle so that you can get to the cause of your struggle. You no longer wish to shed pounds only to gain them all back, so pray for assistance with the cause in order to avoid the symptom of being heavy. This can heal you in every way, but you need to ask for the Truth, and you must be patient.

4. Get quiet and listen. Prayer is a two-way communication, so be still and listen to the guidance that God is giving you. You have to be willing to hear what your Creator is asking and act on this knowledge. It takes practice to understand the messages of the Most High. Sometimes you'll get an obvious response—for example, a thought, picture, or voice may pop into your mind almost instantaneously. Other times, it's much more subtle, such as a sensation of lightness or a shift in consciousness. After a while, you'll start to trust that your prayers are always answered, even if it happens in a way that you don't expect or the timing isn't what you thought it would be.

5. Use positive affirmations that are charged with emotion. These statements are declaring your intentions to the Universe and expressing your willingness and strong desire to live in a new way. Here are some examples:

- *God's strength is within me now.*
- *I am drawn to healthy foods.*
- *My eating habits are easily changing for the better.*
- *My Creator's love is ever-present and strengthening me.*
- *I can be still and listen to the Divine voice.*
- *The Almighty is my guide and my helper.*
- *My body is a holy vessel.*
- *My life is a gift from God.*

6. Use your imagination. See, feel, and know the truth of these statements at every level of your being; and mentally experience how good these new behaviors feel. Affirm that your prayers are being answered and that these shifts are occurring now. As you step into this new reality, realize that this is God's plan for you. Everything that you've been through has brought you to where you're willing to accept your greater good. Through your healing, you'll become a positive force for everyone around you.

7. Give thanks for all that you've been given. Finding this book and having the strength to make a new choice is one such blessing. Express appreciation for your transformation as if it's already happened. Remember all the abundance in your life, and praise God from your heart with gratitude. A prayer of thanksgiving opens the door for more blessings.

With these principles in mind, let's get started on the exercise (there's no need to record it):

Place your hand on your chest, consciously set the intention to drop away from your mental chatter, and focus on your heart as a doorway to the Divine. Visualize a beautiful, fragrant rose blossoming within you, and remember that God's grace can only flow through an open heart.

Imagine yourself breathing in and out of the center of your upper chest. To truly access this place, you must drop your consciousness to it. Imagine two nostrils there and the name of God written in light.

If you have any difficulty with this, try physically putting your head down and bowing to yourself. This movement may help you achieve a state of reverence as you speak to God. Picture a holy jewel at your core; this gem is your own unique expression of a Higher Power here on Earth.

Drop any expectations you may have that in order to be "spiritual," you mustn't have any faults. You're a heavenly being who's having a human experience, and your animal nature comes from your Creator. With intention and grace, you can offer that part of you back to your Source to be transformed into a Higher State—but the pace at which you travel isn't up to you. The only choice you have is your willingness; the rest is in the hands of God. You're only asked to be patient and have faith.

Express your humble appreciation and your sincere desire to be of service. Recognize that the fastest way to grow is through gratitude and the desire to help, love, and teach others what you've been given— in other words, you can only receive more of what you pass on. Like a single candle that can light an infinite number of others without losing its flame, you were placed here to shine for whoever is placed on your path.

Tell God how stuck you feel when it comes to eating nutritious food and maintaining a healthy weight. Ask to be shown a new way and to be given the strength and courage to live it; then take the time to be quiet and let the Lord hold you. It's a subtle feeling, but if you turn your focus within, you'll feel the safety and protection.

Envision your prayer emanating from your heart, not your head. Imagine that your deepest essence has a voice and that your words are being spoken from under your hand (which is resting high on your chest).

Open up to receive the blessings that will automatically come to you; listen and accept what you're being given. In the same way that you might stretch your awareness to hear beautiful music that was coming from the next room, reach out to experience a higher reality, even if you don't perceive it yet. Positive expectancy is the key.

Exercise 24: Prayer to Forgive Yourself

If you're having difficulty forgiving yourself, personal prayer can help you create lasting change. Free yourself from any blame, and bask in compassion and mercy. It takes great courage to face yourself this way, so really acknowledge your commitment to life and health.

The following prayer will help you open yourself to Divine forgiveness; feel free to modify it to reflect your own beliefs about your Higher Power (there's no need to record it):

Dear Lord, I'm so sorry for how I've treated my body. I regret all the years that I used food for comfort when life got difficult, rather than turning to You.

I ask for forgiveness and for Your help in completely transforming the way that I think about myself and eating. Please show me specifically which behaviors I need to change and how to do so. I seek the wisdom to know which foods are best for me (and which are harmful), and the strength to act on what I'm shown. Thank you so much.

I'm sorry for all the ways I haven't listened to You. Turn my heart and mind to You and protect me from the voices that sabotage me. Please fill me with Your strength, because I want to change my ways and live in the highest way possible. I wish to truly honor this miraculous body that You've given me. Thank You.

DOES PRAYER REALLY WORK?

Can you be sure that prayer will help you achieve the results you want? Well, what do you have to lose? What has all your hard work and sincere effort to diet and exercise—without seeking help from your Higher Power—amounted to? Think about how much of your life you've already devoted to these efforts . . . and how much longer you'll continue to do so.

You need to surrender your conventional ideas of what you should do and what it will take for you to be thin. Accept the fact that you're helpless in this area of your life and need assistance from a greater Source. I suggest that you put your faith in your Creator, using prayer and the six steps of the Right Weigh program. As you pray for personal change and guidance on how to follow through, you'll learn what actions you need to take. And when you begin to trust what you're shown and make a commitment to act on it, you'll begin to see new results in your life.

Maybe praying seems too simple and ordinary to be of any great use. Remember: It doesn't preclude action. By speaking with God, you'll be guided to the actions that will lead you to the result you desire rather than struggling in desperation. When you act from the deeper parts of yourself—from your heart and soul's sincere longing to do what you've been shown in prayer—everything will start to flow easily. You won't have to force yourself to exercise or eat "diet" food. Instead, you'll naturally begin to make choices that will lead to health and achieving your ideal weight.

God provides an underlying order to the chaos of life. As you come to recognize this, you'll begin to trust that everything, even your most painful experiences, exists or came about in order to help you manifest something new and beautiful in your life.

You're so much more than your limited body and intellectual capacity. My prayer for you is that through this program you'll not only achieve a body that you can feel comfortable in and happy with, but that you'll also come to see and know that every thought you have is a prayer. In every single moment and with every breath you take, you can make new choices, which is evidence of just how much your Creator loves you. What you do with this knowledge is up to you. . . .

ASKING GOD FOR HELP

There's a good chance that you already pray, since so many people claim that they do. I suggest that you make a commitment to do so regularly with intention and focus—to trust that God wants you to have what you long for and to be free from the past. These exercises will teach you to enter into this Divine conversation with passion, not passively or in a rote way. You'll be transformed to the extent that you do it consistently, sincerely, and with the willingness to apply what you receive to your daily life.

If you only brushed your teeth when you had a toothache, for example, it would be better than not cleaning them at all, but it wouldn't bring about a favorable result for your mouth. It's the same thing with sporadic, rote, or distracted prayer. But through regular, focused effort, you'll begin to unfold into your innate higher potential, just as the sun and the rain take an ordinary flower bulb and allow it to become the magnificent blossom it was always meant to be.

If you're unsure about taking the time to commune with your Source, think about the alternative: How much more pain can you endure in this area of your life? How much more money, time, and energy are you willing to commit to your obsessions about your weight and addiction to food? When you finally pray from a place of supplication and humility and show God your weakness, you'll give permission for Divine strength to flow into every pore of your being.

Now when I use the term *weakness,* I'm not implying that you're less than anyone else. The ego likes to feel strong and powerful in the world and convince itself that it's invincible. If it succeeds in convincing others of its greatness through material success, physical beauty, intelligence, or accomplishment—or even by inflicting pain on others—it feels successful. But the truth is that despite what the ego says, we're inherently weak underneath it all. We have no control over whether we'll still be breathing five minutes from now; we're here only by the grace of the Universal Life Force.

I'm not talking about a God Whom many religious groups have used throughout time as a vehicle to inflict their own agenda on the human race. I mean a loving, compassionate Force that, behind all the drama we've created, is holding each and every one of us. When you're humble and call on this Power when you feel weak, you'll be filled with strength every time.

All it takes is practice, commitment, and a willingness to say, "I have nothing to lose. I'll give it a try." So if your inner voices (and perhaps the outer voices of friends or family members) are saying to you: "What?! You're on another diet? How long is that going to last? Why don't you just give up? Eat!" you'll be shown how to bring your awareness to these reactions and bathe them in kindness and love.

Living in the light of the Divine, you'll continue to move toward all that you most desire as you complete the six steps of the Right Weigh program. All that remains is to review some tips for keeping these principles alive in your heart.

●●●●●●

CHAPTER ELEVEN

Commit to Using the Techniques

As you continue making progress toward your dreams, remember that you must make yourself a priority in your own life. Figure out how long it will take you to do the exercises that help you the most, plus your personal prayer time, and write it all down in your calendar as appointments not to be missed. If you don't honor yourself, you'll spend your life fulfilling everyone else's goals for you—and where will that leave you? When you finally decide to put yourself first, you'll realize that it isn't selfish. In fact, it's easier for you to give to those you love and care about when you're healthy, happy, and fulfilled.

Dealing with Resistance

As you work this program and move forward, you'll come up against resistance from within and outside of yourself. Even if your loved ones are skeptical at first, don't let that deter you. Give them time to adjust to the changes you're making.

After so many years of suffering, you finally have the tools to make your vision real, so don't look back. People may try to talk you out of self-hypnosis, Remembrance, or prayer, telling you that it's a waste of time. You don't have to justify your actions or get upset with them. Just stay present in your body, and if you choose, you can share what you've discovered and why you're committed to personal growth and continuing with these practices. Simply speak from your own experience. If they have trouble supporting you, give them love and mercy, and have faith in their ability to make the adjustment.

If you're still unsure whether you're deriving any benefit from the exercises, that's okay, too. As long as you know in your heart that you're committed to this program and have faith that you can reach your goal with the help of your internal Source, that's all that matters.

If you experience resistance from within, pray for the inner fortitude you need. Remember that the greatest aid you're getting is from the inside, deep within your soul and spirit. You see, those who question you on the outside are mirroring your own doubts. When you reaffirm your choice to take the higher road and are very clear about this within your own being, that outer opposition will drop away as well. Then it will become much easier to be compassionate toward your loved ones, who are struggling to accept your changes.

Getting Back on Track

It's natural to feel skeptical as you continue working with the six steps. Rest assured that the voices of doubt and negativity *will* creep in—and that they serve a purpose. They're there to test you to see how committed you are to making higher choices consistently, especially in the face of difficulty, so be ready. Sometimes they'll well up within you, and often they'll come from those you care about the most. But now you know how to contain, challenge, and transform these challenges without being sucked in. Always remember that you know where you're going, no matter how off course you may feel in the moment.

I highly recommend that you find a friend to travel this path with you or start a Right Weigh support group with a few other people so that you can assist each other in getting back to your essential nature. Community can be so helpful when you begin to walk a road that isn't necessarily the most well-worn path. It's easy to find plenty of people to commiserate with when you're down, but it can be immensely beneficial to have companions who also long to find freedom from their suffering. You can practice doing the exercises together. If you can't find anyone in your area, you can write to me and perhaps I can put you in touch with someone you can work with over the telephone. You can reach me through my Website: **www.easywillpower.com**.

Keeping the Momentum

To keep on making headway, it's crucial that you write down your weight-loss strategy—that is, the actions you're going to take to make your dreams a reality. Making that commitment to yourself will help you keep going forward. If you feel moved to continue practicing the exercises in Part II beyond the initial 40 days, by all means do so. Why would you stop using such powerful tools once you've realized the benefits you can gain from them?

There's so much temptation to go outside yourself in this world, but stay steadfast and continue your journey inward. There's no end to the treasures inside you, and when you discover that, your search for inner peace will be over. Once you know where to look, you can make your vision a reality.

The tools you've acquired in this book can improve your life in so many ways that it truly is a miracle. Keep up the momentum you've established with your hard work and sincere desire for a better life. You deserve all of the beautiful offerings to be had in this world. You're now open to receiving these gifts and are willing to cleanse the old wounds that prevent your growth, and you have the techniques to make it happen.

There's no limit to where this path can take you—certainly well beyond simply having the body that you so desperately wish to have. Stay focused and you can realize your vision for your life. And most important, always give thanks for the journey and all that you've been taught along the way.

I hope that out of the array of exercises presented here, you found some that resonated for you. Although many people get great results almost immediately, others need to practice for a while before they notice any effect. If you haven't already begun the program, gather the tools you'll need (a journal, a tape recorder and tapes, index cards, and sticky notes) and get started today. Please don't procrastinate.

If you're already on your way but have doubts about the road ahead, just read the motivation list that you made in Step 1. Think about the pleasure of being healthy, slender, energetic, fit, and in control, as opposed to the pain of keeping things as they are. Know that freedom from addiction, bingeing, and feeling unhealthy does await you. In fact, by continuing with the techniques you've learned in this book, you'll experience freedom in more areas of your life than you can possibly imagine.

Coming from the Heart

In order to work the Right Weigh program, you can't just read these ideas and hope that your goals will manifest. When you stay in your head in that way, it's easy to get caught in the futile process of deciding whether or not you believe in a Higher Power. Instead, I encourage you to drop your focus to your heart and receive all the love that your Creator is making available with every breath. It doesn't matter if you've never consciously been in touch with that compassion before. If you have faith that it's there and act as if it were, new worlds of joy and peace will open up for you.

You may find yourself humbly watching the process of your life transforming, the way you might stand in awe at the sight of a magnificent vista in nature or a baby being born. Your task is to put your focus on the greater perspective and continually decide to follow it.

Once you acknowledge that this Force not only exists, but that you're connected to it through your heart, it's much easier to make an inner commitment to allow this Source to lead you. You'll come to realize that only by aligning with Divine love can you ever come to know true happiness and win the battle with your weight forever.

Surrender to this Higher Power by staying connected to your heart with prayer, awareness, and the practice of Remembrance. As you go through this process, you'll begin to ask your inner wisdom for guidance before you take action and wait until you hear, feel, or just know the answer.

I encourage you to let the light within your soul guide you every step of the way, no matter what you're experiencing in the outer world. In time, your life circumstances will change, and you'll begin to realize your goals. You only need to stay steadfast on the journey.

A New Awareness

One day you might realize that you no longer crave certain dishes, and it will be easier to leave some of your meal on your plate. You may start to look forward to riding your bike, walking, or incorporating some other new activity into your routine. As you get more in touch with your physical self, it will become even clearer which foods support you and which ones bring you heartache. You'll happily give up a temporary desire for the long-term satisfaction of a healthy and vibrant life; and you'll find yourself enjoying simply breathing, moving your body, and feeling your stomach slightly empty. You won't be as tired anymore, or as angry. What a gift it will be to know that you've changed! You'll look back in awe and see the path you've walked, knowing that every step—even the most painful—has helped you grow into the person you are today.

The reality is that you're already lovely, but you just need to realize it. Sometimes you forget to see all the inner and outer beauty that you carry. You think that you need to change, but the truth is that you just need to make some adjustments in the way you think about yourself, food, and the quality of your life. You *can* break through the limitations that have kept you trapped, and experience boundless joy and energy. Not only will your weight drop, but you'll also enjoy more peace than you ever thought possible.

When you go digging for this gold, please know that the only place to look is in your heart, and if you haven't yet found these riches, it simply means that you need to be patient and go deeper. The treasure you seek is truly inside you, and your desire for a healthy body that looks and feels great will motivate you to find it.

My prayer for you is that this book will serve as your guide and your teacher, and leave you not only inspired but absolutely committed to tuning in to that higher station of Divine love and wisdom within your own being. May you enjoy and gain insight from every step of this journey, and may your life be filled with blessings and unlimited possibilities for happiness.

ACKNOWLEDGMENTS

I have so much gratitude to all the people who helped me write and publish this book. First and foremost, I want to thank my devoted husband, Barry, who has always been there to support me in every way. I'm so grateful for his love and unending support, which has helped me grow and gave me a constant source of strength. My angelic daughters, Crystal and Jessie, have been such a deep well of love and faith for me. Their love never ceases to inspire me.

Thank you to Jill Kramer and Shannon Littrell of Hay House who have been a pleasure to work with, and whose feedback has been invaluable. I also wish to thank Hay House for the gift of publishing this book for me.

I had the privilege of working with an incredibly wise and creative editor—Nancy Peske. Her knowledge and expert advice made the project fun for me as well as an incredible learning experience. In addition, her warmth and friendship during the process was much appreciated.

I want to offer my deepest thanks to my longtime friend Lynda Luppino, who encouraged me from day one to follow my heart and gave me the help I needed to pursue my dreams.

My literary agent, Linda Konner, has been an incredible source of encouragement and assistance throughout the process, and I'm very appreciative of her down-to-earth support and positive approach.

I'm very appreciative of the love and support from all my friends and family. Most of all, I want to thank my wonderful mother, Lore Prag, who has always believed in and encouraged me and been there for me in every way. My sisters, Nurit and Shula, have added a richness to my life. I especially want to thank Nurit for all of her valuable contributions.

Also, I'm very grateful to my loving father and mother-in-law, Arthur and Evelyn Greenberg, as well as all my brothers- and sisters-in-law for their support—with a special thank you to Joyce and Craig Parsley and Paula Greenberg, who touched me deeply by taking the time to give me some very valuable feedback.

I'm so thankful to my friends who were by my side helping and encouraging me during the creation of *The Right Weigh.* A special thank you to Ellen Tishman, Ann Kingsbury, Denise Marsico, Polly Katz, Kathie Daniel, Merry Berger, and Eileen Calarco for their profound gifts. I'll always have deep appreciation for Nathan Greenberg, whose generosity made it possible for me to sit down and begin the creation of this book.

A warm thank you to the hearts who have significantly lightened my life: Pat Bayer, Barbara Englehardt, Diana Cavallo, Vaishnavii Lewis, Pauline Dixon, and Jolene Mills.

I'm very grateful to the many thousands of people who attended my Wellness Seminar for weight loss over the past 17 years, giving me the opportunity to share what I've learned over time and help them reach their weight goals. It was only through working with these sincere people and seeing their longing for a road map to permanent weight loss that I've been inspired to write this book and share what I've been given to help others not only lose weight, but also live in health and happiness.

Thank you to my magnificent teachers who were always there for me along the way. I offer a special thanks to Dr. Robert Jaffe, who helped make this book possible in many ways—most of all by teaching me the power of the love in my deep heart. I want to thank the many wonderful teachers I've been blessed with throughout my life, most recently at the University of Spiritual Studies and Sufism, including Salima Adelstein, Dr. John Laird, Nura Laird, Paul Werner, Sabura Tierney, Ryhana Rae, Jim Keeley, Jeff Bronner, Mark Silver, Adam and Laila Cayce, Aisha and Salih Cotten, Gregory Lee, Na'ama McCreedy, and Khadija Gigliotti. Their love, wisdom, guidance, and life-changing teachings helped me embrace new possibilities. I also want to thank the many wonderful people who stepped in to offer a contribution, with a special thanks to Laila Brady and Dr. Carolyn Dixon for their generosity of spirit.

Finally, I wish to express deep thanks for all my dear friends and classmates, especially Donna Bartholomew, Karen Ball, Christine Armata, Claude Mann, Amy Carpentieri, Raina Stinson, and Marcia Sheline, who have offered me a well of support as I undertook this project. Most of all, I wish to thank my Guide, Sidi, whose heart is an ocean of the deep love and mercy for all of humanity.

Rena Greenberg has been the director of Wellness Seminars, Inc., since 1990. She has successfully conducted weight-control conferences for major organizations such as Walt Disney World, Busch Gardens, AT&T, and Home Depot, as well as in over 70 hospitals throughout New York, Florida, Michigan, and Ohio. Since 1989, she's helped more than 100,000 people achieve their weight goals.

Rena is a graduate of City University of New York with a degree in biopsychology. She's a certified hypnotherapist through the National Guild of Hypnotists, as well as a nationally certified biofeedback therapist. Rena has appeared on numerous radio and television programs, and she continues to speak on a regular basis about weight loss to large audiences throughout Florida and Michigan.

Website: **www.easywillpower.com**

We hope you enjoyed this Hay House book.
If you'd like to receive a free catalog featuring additional
Hay House books and products, or if you'd like information
about the Hay Foundation, please contact:

Hay House, Inc.
P.O. Box 5100
Carlsbad, CA 92018-5100

(760) 431-7695 or **(800) 654-5126**
(760) 431-6948 (fax) or **(800) 650-5115 (fax)**
www.hayhouse.com • www.hayfoundation.org

Published and distributed in Australia by: Hay House Australia Pty. Ltd.
18/36 Ralph St. • Alexandria NSW 2015 • *Phone:* 612-9669-4299 •
Fax: 612-9669-4144 • www.hayhouse.com.au

Published and distributed in the United Kingdom by: Hay House UK, Ltd.
Unit 62, Canalot Studios • 222 Kensal Rd., London W10 5BN •
Phone: 44-20-8962-1230 • *Fax:* 44-20-8962-1239 • www.hayhouse.co.uk

Published and distributed in the Republic of South Africa by: Hay House
SA (Pty), Ltd., P.O. Box 990, Witkoppen 2068 • *Phone/Fax:* 27-11-706-6612
• orders@psdprom.co.za

Distributed in Canada by: Raincoast • 9050 Shaughnessy St.,
Vancouver, B.C. V6P 6E5 • *Phone:* (604) 323-7100 • *Fax:* (604) 323-2600

Tune in to **www.hayhouseradio.com**™ for the best in inspirational
talk radio featuring top Hay House authors! And, sign up via the
Hay House USA Website to receive the Hay House online newsletter and
stay informed about what's going on with your favorite authors. You'll
receive bimonthly announcements about: Discounts and Offers, Special
Events, Product Highlights, Free Excerpts, Giveaways, and more!
www.hayhouse.com